# THE SOUL OF BEAUTY

# THE SOUL OF BEAUTY

## A Psychological Investigation of Appearance

Ronald Schenk

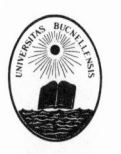

Lewisburg
Bucknell University Press
London and Toronto: Associated University Presses

Associated University Presses
440 Forsgate Drive
Cranbury, NJ 08512

Associated University Presses
25 Sicilian Avenue
London WC1A 2QH, England

Associated University Presses
P.O. Box 39, Clarkson Pstl. Stn.
Mississauga, Ontario,
L5J 3X9 Canada


The paper used in this publication meets the requirements
of the American National Standard for Permanence of Paper
for Printed Library Materials Z39.48-1984.


Library of Congress Cataloging-in-Publication Data

Schenk, Ronald, 1944–
     The soul of beauty : a psychological investigation of appearance /
Ronald Schenk.
        p.   cm.
     Includes bibliographical references and index.
     ISBN 0-8387-5214-4 (alk. paper)
     1. Aesthetics—Psychological aspects—History.   2. Psychology and
philosophy—History.   I. Title.
BH301.P78S34   1992
150'.1—dc20                                                        91-55125
                                                                        CIP


PRINTED IN THE UNITED STATES OF AMERICA

# CONTENTS

*To Charlotte*

# ILLUSTRATIONS

# FOREWORD

This is an accomplished work, written in the tradition of James Hillman and J. H. van den Berg, with a complex but coherent argument
that is both original and persuasive. It addresses modern psychology
and its dilemma, first noted by phenomenologists, perhaps, but elaborated in a Jungian way by Hillman. Psychology is an awkward step-
child of the modern age, fitting neither the scientific world of material
reality and overt action nor the spiritual world of meaning and motive,
consciousness and perception. The split between the material and
spiritual worlds, beginning in Greek thought, eventually culminates in
the modern predicament of psychology.

The split suggests a prior unity to which we can return. Indeed
psychology, especially in the practice of psychotherapy, already does so
daily, but without a legitimate status in the world of science. It dangles
between science and art, material reality and human perception, main-
taining itself without a footing in either world by depending on the
mere suffering of humanity. This suffering does not, as human existence itself does not, allow itself to be reduced either to the physical
world of science nor to the transcendental world of meaning. (Indeed,
it is exactly this split that is the suffering of "modern man in search of a
soul," to use Jung's phrase.) Therefore, that unity which we might
recover from the ancients, we already have, are, and live daily.

Schenk's essay tries to help us to see this prior unity clearly by
reviewing our understanding of beauty, which is neither "subjective"
(in the eye of the beholder and irrelevant to what things really are and
mean) nor "objective" (grasped through the categories of scientific
reality). Beauty is neither; it is both; or, more precisely, it is prior to this
bifurcation. Our experience of beauty at once engages us in both
worlds. Our experience of beauty moves us both physically and spiritually. So does psychology.

# PART ONE: BEAUTY AS APPEARANCE

## CHAPTER 1. APHRODITE

> To recover the psychological value of beauty, we would need to restore the "metaphysical dignity" it held for the Greeks. This would require entering into the world of Aphrodite, the divine personification of beauty. (p. 37)

Aphrodite is beauty in herself; she refers to nothing beyond herself; she personifies beauty. The radiance of this beauty weds the erotic and the sacred—matter and ideality, animality and spirit. Furthermore, Aphrodite has a dark side; having given birth to terror and fear, she has such capabilities for us. But most important, what appears, her beauty, is her essence; depth lies on the surface, and we are moved both by her particularity and her universality.

## CHAPTER 2. BEAUTY AS LIGHT

The Neoplatonic tradition provides the foundation for a psychological paradigm of beauty. The author leads the reader through discussions of several aspects of this paradigm.

Beauty and Order. Plato's writing often suggests that the transcendent realm is purely ideal and that material things, by contrast, are degraded and deprived. Certainly, much Christian appropriation of Plato interprets him this way, and the Greek sense of "cosmic piety" makes this persuasive. However, Plotinus and Ficino interpreted Plato such that the spiritual center of the universe (not a separate transcendental realm) permeates the concentric layers of reality, all the way to materiality. Armstrong more recently follows this line of interpretation, which connects concrete beauty in material things to the higher principle of beauty.

This non-Christian reading of Plato is much more useful for psychology, and Schenk notes that Hillman is among many who take it. It makes it possible for image (perception as meaning) to be grounded in both the spiritual realm (the principle of beauty) and matter (things of the world). And it obviates the traditional split between the realms that plagues psychology today.

Beauty as Mediator. For Plato, of all the forms, only Beauty is visible. Only beauty enables the Divine to manifest itself. Consciousness perceives through the shining forth of beauty in things, and only beauty enables perception to take place.

> The coporeal needs the divine as its source and light. The divine needs the corporeal through which to manifest itself. (p. 51)

For Plotinus, this also becomes the formula for the relation of particular to universal. Seeing the universal in the particular and the
divine in the corporeal is reminiscent of the Renaissance, as opposed to
the medieval sensibility that builds on the transcendent reading of
hierarchy.

LOVE.

> Beauty moves the soul, and the soul's attitude toward beauty is one of
> passion. (p. 54)
> How different the sense of aesthetic perception as passionate, painful
> desire is from the notion in the subjectivist paradigm where aesthetic
> perception is "disinterested" and accompanied only by the feeling of plea-
> sure. (p. 55)

BEAUTY IN PERCEPTION: Making and Knowing.

> My reading of Plato is that the vision of beauty joins the soul with
> appearance in a conjunction of love, and in the perceiving, image is both
> created and revealed (p. 57)
> The images of impassioned movement and creativity in Plato and
> Plotinus in relation to the aesthetic vision provides for a sense of action in
> seeing. The action is contemplative rather than overt and has a loving
> quality rather than one of control. The aesthetic vision, then, would not
> only honor but care for appearance, considering perception and the images
> of its own creation as one and the same. (p. 58)

BEAUTY AND KNOWLEDGE. Schenk has been aiming toward this topic
and owes readers a finale, for if he is to argue for the possibility of
another way of interpreting human experience, he will have to overcome the objections of modern science, which never tires of reminding
us of the error of perception. Beauty, thus, will have to be reclaimed
from the dustbin of subjectivity and unreliability. Beauty will have to
yield knowledge.

Not surprisingly, Heidegger is a key to the finale, for Heidegger's
reinterpretation of Greek thought remains one of the twentieth century's great challenges. I shall skip several steps in this argument.

> In sum, earthly perceptions, reminding the soul of the divine forms through
> their beauty, are gathered together in the service of the *eidos* that is akin to
> the divine form. These perceptions are shaped into image through the
> organizing influence of the *eidos*. The image brings about the memory of the
> truth of these perceptions. Acquisition of knowledge, then, is a matter of
> memory through beauty. (p. 59)

THE AESTHETICS OF LIGHT: The Many and the One. Plotinus, Dionysius, Ficino, and Gadamer take the reader to the conflict of multiperspectival consciousness versus the logocentric consciousness of singular perspective. The attempt here is to honor the particularity of each perception by relativizing singular consciousness.

BEAUTY AND THE ONE: Unity, Goodness, and Being. The Neoplatonic tradition attempts to establish that beauty, as the perception of ap-pearance, is the foundation of consciousness and thus the ground of being.

Although Schenk is attempting to elaborate a truly psychological paradigm in all of its depth and complexity, these last two sections do not, as does the sequence of previous sections, deal with issues necessary to the argument. I do, however, find the final brief section luminous:

> Image both reveals and conceals, contains both truth and deceit. . . . If it is image or light or appearance or beauty that constitutes the primary realm of human experience or that establishes the ground of truth's possibility or that makes being manifest, then we live *in* image, appearance, light, or beauty and therefore can't know it. . . . it is image, appearance, light, and beauty that are seeing *through* us. Ultimately, what unites us is not our seeing, but that which we can't see, because it makes consciousness possible in the first place. Like the dying Goethe, we want "more light," but paradoxically, it is in the darkness that we find our home. (pp. 67–68)

# PART TWO: BEAUTY AS INTERIOR EXPERIENCE

## CHAPTER 3. APHRODITE REFUSED

> My purpose in this chapter will not be to devalue spirit or concept, but to indicate how spirit and reason in the service of spirit can lead to a devaluing of appearance. (p. 71)

Augustine is central, as is the entire Christian emphasis on heavenly goodness and earthly depravity. Augustine's reading of Genesis, that free will is overcome by the ravages of sexuality and original sin, which in turn necessitates control of humanity by the Church or the state, echoes an earlier turning by the apostle Paul away from works in the world, and toward inner belief and piety. This move seems to overcome the dangers of the deceptions of "mere" appearance, and to assure certainty amidst the fickleness of bodily vulnerability.

Aphrodite becomes a demon. Schenk offers a selection of Christian degradations of Greek polytheism and ancient culture. So dedicated to the Heavenly Father were the Christians that not only sexuality but

also worldly appearance in general were deemed a threat and branded as evil. The intricate controversies about icons in the eighth and ninth centuries, which also express the split between Eastern and European branches of Christianity, put the moral, as well as the metaphysical, status of appearance at stake.

Protestantism, the patriarchal degradation of women, the valuation of reason over imagination by Milton—these are among the data Schenk marshals to present a different paradigm of beauty—one of reason, interiority, spirituality, and certainty—that replaces the pas-sionate corporeality of Aphrodite.

## CHAPTER 4. PROPORTION: BEAUTY AS MEASURE

From spirit Schenk moves to concept, specifically the concept of proportion. Proportion is quantitative, appreciated spiritually, ab-stractly, rather than corporeally. Plato, following Pythagoras, organ-ized his notion of man's relation to the ideal through the concept of proportion. Likewise, Augustine equated beauty with number, liberating it from pagan precursors and defending it with a spiritual identifica-tion. To the extent that beauty is good, it is associated proportionately through number with a transcendent God and grasped only spiritually (rationally and in faith), not sensually. The most perfect geometric figure thus becomes the single point, perfectly centered and unified. The gain for spiritual certitude that proportion offers, however, comes at a loss to the perspective of soul, which values the sensuous par-ticularity of the world.

> When beauty is seen as measure, particular phenomena are seen as frag-mented and become undervalued in themselves. Proportion becomes the mode of perception that is most comfortable because it allows for a sense of control through number and an alignment with the divine. By contrast, when beauty is seen in appearance, the fragment becomes a center in itself. Those phenomena that are skewed and grotesque from a centristic stand-point become rich in inherent value when seen in terms of their ap-pearance.
>
> In summary, although proportion gives rise to a sense of certainty and order, it also favors number over appearance, the unity of numerical system over the inherent value of the particular, and moves consciousness away from an intimate connection with the world. (p. 89)

## CHAPTER 5. LINEAR PERSPECTIVE

This chapter is historical in nature because it deals with a development in the paradigm of beauty as an inner phenomenon during the Renaissance. The development has to do with the transformation of proportion as a

metaphysical system into its literalization as a methodology of representation, namely, linear perspective. In this transformation, the metaphysics of
relating parts to a center developed into a method of depicting the natural
world. . . . Linear perspective, like the concept of proportion upon which it
is based, reflects a need for control, exactitude of measure, stability, and the
security of order. (p. 90)

This quotation lays out ambitious claims. The argument cannot be a
simple one, and this is not an easy argument to follow. First, one notes
that the Renaissance was a time when the transcendental orientation
of the medieval period was overcome and replaced by a worldly and
human centered orientation. Schenk speaks here of a "discovery of the
world" that nevertheless continued to see the divine and the natural as
permeating one another. Mathematics plays an important role:

The theoretical space of the mathematician, the infinite space of the
theologian, and physical space came to be one and the same. Therefore,
mathematics came to be seen as the means for alignment with God. (p. 92)

Linear perspective is, in Schenk's view, more than a technical matter
for painters. It is the format within which human centered perception
can maintain its divine inspiration and avoid debauching into the
depravity of sensual orientation. This temptation necessitates control,
as if the Augustinian background were never surpassed.

The importance of the center in the metaphysics of proportion and the
technique of linear perspective reflects a logocentric philosophical and
moral priority in the Western mind. As Samuel Edgerton asserts, "Europeans came more and more to believe that things planned or seen from a
central viewpoint had greater monumentality and moral authority than
those which were not.) (p. 96)
    In sum, the identification with God that comes with the fixed, centristic
view of linear perspective serves a need for order, control, and certainty.
Singularity of vision imparts the certainty of the way or the truth. . . .
With linear perspective, the subject achives a sense of control over experience. The world becomes something to be manipulated or something that
potentially can be used or consumed. (p. 98)

Appearance itself becomes a by-product of this orientation, instead of
the other way around. Making the world man's object instead of God's,
in this century, is what Max Weber called the "disenchantment of the
world."

It is in the Renaissance that light begins to die out, the universe starts to
turn inward into the mind of human beings, and the world becomes an

object to be measured. Out of this mentality, in the Enlightenment of the eighteenth century, aesthetics as the science of taste is born. Beauty becomes subjectivized and subordinate, separated from the fundaments of power, necessity, truth, good, and being, which it inhabits in the paradigm of beauty as appearance. (p. 100)

## CHAPTER 6. THE SUBJECTIVIZATION OF BEAUTY

Descartes's *cogito ergo sum* reinforces all these trends with philo-sophical certainty centered in human subjectivity. But the center of the subjectivization of beauty was in the British aesthetic phi-losophers. Through Shaftsbury, Hutchinson, Addison, Burke, Alison, and Hume, the author traces the progressive loss of the "light" of the ancients.

> When beauty is subjective, one might say, the world no longer offers itself forth to be known through direct apprehension. Instead, truth is estab-lished by perception of the world through the grid of logic and abstract concepts. (p. 108)

Schenk then turns to Kant, whose philosophy presumably saved Western thought from disappearance into the subject. There are sev-eral readings of Kant, and Schenk prefers Heidegger's interpretation, which highlights the notion that perception without desire needn't be mere passive reception but rather a matter of "letting things be." Like knowledge, beauty is grasped by a universal archetype, it is communi-cable, links subject and object, and is congruent with the good. How-ever, the British influence is also present in Kant, and these themes are usually emphasized in modern interpretations.

In conclusion:

> In the paradigm of beauty as an internal phenomenon of mind, truth is held to lie in number, beauty becomes a notion of symmetry and wholeness, and aesthetics becomes a separate discipline of perception through feeling. As aesthetics becomes separated from truth, imagination and feeling be-come estranged from cognition, and the latter takes on the quality of certainty. Human sciences turn to methodology for understanding; beauty becomes literalized in art; educated consciousness becomes necessary for aesthetic perception; creativity becomes a personal matter; and art falls into the domain of genius. Beauty is now depotentiated, no longer associated with truth, utility, action, and an inherent faith in appearance. (p. 116)

## PART THREE: THE RETURN OF AESTHETICS IN CONTEMPORARY PSYCHOLOGY

### CHAPTER 7. IMAGE IN DEPTH PSYCHOLOGY

> The orientation of the first section was that beauty, when seen psycho-
> logically, is the ground of everyday being and knowing. In the final section,
> I would like to give an account of the recovery of this sense of beauty
> through depth psychology, focusing particularly on Jung's later thought and
> psychotherapy as a cultural manifestation of the aesthetic mode. Finally, I
> attempt to formulate an aesthetic psychology based upon the imaginal
> psychology of James Hillman. (p. 119)

Schenk broaches this task through a discussion of two aesthetic
thinkers, Neitzsche and Blake, and argues that they offer two crucial
themes: the value of unmediated perception ("letting things be"), and
the active/creative nature of such nonconceptual human perception.

Nietzsche's discussion of Dionysion and Apollonian modes of experience portrays the human reliance on the order of Apollonian concepts,
even as they distort and falsify the "original mass of similes and
percepts pouring forth as a fiery liquid out of the primal faculty of
human fancy," to use Nietzsche's words (p. 121). Truth and life belong
to aesthetic experience, not mediated by the trivial pleasures of refined
delicacy, but engulfed by the storms of perception that dares to face the
world as it presents itself, full of motion, noise, and unpredictability. It
is in this experience that humanity is creative and hence most human.

Blake also singles out the creative imagination as what saves us from
a fallen and false world. "This does not mean that only the artist can
be redeemed, but that all of redeemed life follows the principles of the
artistic process of creative imagination" (p. 122).

With Nietzsche and Blake, there is a shift from "light" to "image"
as the name for and locus of the link between humanity and world,
experience and meaning, perception and truth; this name emerges in
contemporary psychology.

The author begins his discussion of image in contemporary psychology with Freud, Jung's precursor and teacher, who also was basically
modern in his view of the image as "archaic," an expression of the
unconscious, regressive and primitive, in contrast to the secondary
process and reality principle of intellection, which governs understanding. Dreams and images are merely a means to information and
are not information in themselves.

This attitude prefigured Jung, who, early in his thought, displayed a
distinct mistrust of image and sought to get beyond the image to
meaning. But by the time of his symbolic and alchemical writings,

Jung's postmodern sensibilities show through in passages like the
following: "Image and meaning are identical and as the first takes
shape, the latter becomes clear. Actually the pattern needs no interpretation; it portrays its own meaning." This violates Freud and moder-
nity. Meaning is grounded in the image, and one may interpret
intellection in terms of image rather than the other way around. Truth
is available in image. According to Schenk:

> Appearance itself is all that is necessary when perceived through the
> aesthetic eye unmediated by concept. (p. 131)

This move by Jung has been appreciated before, but it is only in the
context of this book that one sees its importance. If I have a dream of
anima nurturing me, it is an option to say that that image is symbolic of
the reality of my mother and my experience of her. Freud would have
it so. However, Jung asks whether it is not the case that my mother
and my experience of her is symbolic of the basic image of anima, and
that basic image is not only a ground of meaning but also a ground of
reality as I experience it at all. Image thus moves from a symbol to a
ground of meaning, including what is called reality. Schenk is onto
something here.

## CHAPTER 8. BEAUTY AND PSYCHOTHERAPY

Thoughts by Hannah Arendt and Gadamer regarding the Greek
notions of the contemplative life and active life give rise to the idea
that talking in psychotherapy is story telling; it is the making present of
self to self through an action that refers constantly to its origin, oneself.
In this way it is a creative self-manifestation of human reality—self and
world.

This creative self-manifestation is analogous to beauty as a self-
referring appearance. It is the creation of human reality. It is modern
culture's counterpart to political action in the Greek city-state, where
the creation of human reality had a different modus operandi, for it
occurred in a different culture and social milieu. What is commonly
understood in our culture as some kind of quasi-medical cure of disease
can be uncommonly understood in Schenk's terms as human creativity
and self-creativity. That is not a bad re-visioning (to use Hillman's
phrase) of what gets crammed thoughtlessly into a medical metaphor
in modern consciousness.

The clinical examples Schenk offers are those of contemporary
Jungian analysts interested in the interactional field between therapist
and patient. They are suggestive. Nathan Schwartz-Salant, for exam-

ple, focuses on the experiential space of therapist and client and what is between—the scene of the speaking and creating. What is created is talk, of course, but also image. Each "sees" what is happening in the room creatively, and they share their "images," thus creating the room and its action between them, thus creating the reality of the therapy, thus creating the reality of themselves, the very human beings seeing and enacting it. The sharing of images created is heady therapeutic dialogue—intimate, courageous, self-exposing, and self-creative. Any psychotherapist will see this. Nonspecialists will not.

## CHAPTER 9. TOWARD A PSYCHOLOGY OF APPEARANCE

The final chapter reveals the incompleteness of this work. But it looks forward to a future completion; it leads readers to think further. Schenk thinks of the new psychology as addressing our cultural problem, described variously as "Cartesian suspicion of the world," "the subject-object split," and the devaluation of appearance, and hence of beauty, as a way of seeing and being in the world.

> I believe that the recovery of beauty is important as a movement toward healing the wound in the modern psyche caused by the separation of appearance and being. The symptom of this separation, Cartesian doubt of the world, reveals the anxiety of consciousness without a home. Without a sense of dwelling, the modern mind is constantly on a journey, incessantly focused upon the horizon in search of meaning. The purpose of the recovery would be to bring consciousness back to dwelling. When meaning is seen in appearance at hand, then beauty provides a habitat for consciousness. (p. 145)

This description refers to the book; it is hard to grasp apart from the book. But the paragraph also refers to something very easy to understand, or at least easy to identify as something very familiar. It is the cycle of suffering and redemption.

Psychology in the modern world at once lives this cycle and yet has no understanding of it like that presented in this work. Aesthetic psychology is familiar, and yet it is not taught. In fact, the psychology that is taught works against one's ability to do what is necessary.

> The therapist starts with the symptom—the depression, the fear, the physiological malady, the feeling of dis-ease—and sees a god at work in this initial "stuff." . . . The aesthetic psychologist is small-minded, noticing closely the detail of the appearance of things. He or she values and cares for these appearances—the discarded, depleted, abandoned, split-off, frag-

mented, rustic, horrible, vulgar, repulsive, obscene, and perverse—as them'
selves being the dispossessed centers of a certain beauty.

An attitude of shocked wonder takes away the literal eye as the primary
organ of sense. "I see it feelingly," says the blinded, but wisened
Gloucester. . . . The organ of seeing aesthetically would be not so much the
literal eye, but the nose of intuition. The nose knows, Joyce continually
tells us. (p. 146)

Indeed, the vision is incomplete. One reads this book, challenged to
complete it for oneself.

ERNEST KEEN

# ACKNOWLEDGMENTS

I would like to acknowledge my gratitude to the work of James Hillman and Hans-Georg Gadamer as inspiration for this book. I am especially grateful to Dr. Hillman for opening my mind to the life of ideas; in many ways, this work is my attempt to develop a foundation for his formulation of imaginal psychology.

I would like to thank my teachers at the University of Dallas where this work was formulated. Robert Kugelmann has been a source of intellectual stimulation and support throughout my association with him. His open-minded attitude and breadth of thought have been a genuine invitation to psychological inquiry and a model for what is best in the teaching of psychology. Robert Wood acted as both guide and midwife for much of this work. He was immensely helpful, not only in leading me through a forest of philosophical thought, but in suggesting a structure that would allow for the emergence of my own ideas. I am grateful to Robert Romanyshyn for his bringing to my awareness the cultural aspect of psychological life, his vision of multi-disciplinary study as psychological training, and his steadfast loyalty to that vision.

I am very appreciative of the support and advice given to me by Paul Kugler, Andrew Samuels, and Robin Robertson who took the time to read an early draft of the work. My conversations with Tom Moore have been greatly rewarding in generating and clarifying ideas.

I am grateful to the Friends of Jung of Phoenix for their support and for giving me the opportunity to test my ideas in a public forum.

My thanks also to Ardith Gibbon for her help in typing an early complete draft, and to Sandy Cassio for her extremely careful and helpful work in correcting the manuscript and making suggestions.

I would like to express my appreciation to my son, Ashley, my former wife, Tina, my parents, and to my friends for their support, cooperation, tolerance, and emotional nurturance. Finally, I would like to acknowledge my gratitude to my wife, Charlotte Parker for her grace, her care, and her love. These people, who have been close to me during trying times, are true sources of beauty in my life.

Excerpts from the following works have been used by permission of the Faber and Faber and Oxford University Press:

*Plotinus: The Enneads,* translated by Stephen MacKenna. London: Faber and Faber, 1956.

*The Critique of Judgement,* by Emmanuel Kant. Oxford: Oxford University Press, 1952.

# INTRODUCTION

My thinking for this book was initiated by a question from a colleague at a presentation on "The Aesthetics of Arthritis."[1] that I gave to a group of psychotherapists. In that paper, I used the term *aesthetic* to refer to the appearance of phenomena. I suggested that disease is the appearance of a way of being in the world and that to perceive the appearance of the arthritic way of being in its full display was, in itself, therapeutic. After the talk, I was asked the question, "But what do we *do?*" The implication was that to speak of aesthetics does not address the question of effectiveness. The questioner could only think of healing in relation to overt action, not the perception of appearance on the part of the therapist.

I couldn't answer the question to my satisfaction at the time, and my feeling of inadequacy stayed with me. I didn't realize until later that the question came from a way of thinking that was different from mine. The questioner saw only action as affecting the world, while I considered perception itself to be effective. For her, action was different from perception, while for me, perception was a form of action in itself.

After exploring the conflict to some extent, I realized that the difference between our approaches reflected a basic split in Western thought between the life of perception and appearance on the one hand, and the life of practical action and meaning on the other. *Perception* is considered as a passive enterprise, which in and of itself, has no effect on the world. Change is brought about through overt action in the world. *Appearance* is associated with that which is merely superficial, while *meaning* is connected with that which is operating invisibly. To attain meaning, one needs to act to uncover it. I undertook the project of this book in the attempt to bridge the gap between perception and appearance on the one hand, and notions such as meaning and action, to which modern consciousness gives priority, on the other.

If one explores the idea of the perception of appearance, one finds a world of meaning that has been lost by modern consciousness. Hannah Arendt states:

> The world men are born into contains many things, natural and ar-
> tificial, living and dead, transient and sempiternal, all of which have in
> common that they *appear* and hence are meant to be seen, heard, touched,
> tasted and smelled, to be perceived by sentient creatures endowed with the
> appropriate sense organs. . . . In this world which we enter, appearing from
> a nowhere, and from which we disappear into a nowhere, *Being and
> Appearing coincide.*[2]

For Arendt, appearance, to be perceived through the five senses, is the
equivalent of being. We are as we appear and vice versa. There is no
need for proof of existence or depth of meaning beyond simple appearance.

The word *aesthetics* comes from the Greek word for the perception
of appearance, *aisthesis,* meaning "of the senses" or "pertaining to the
perception of things." It is connected to the Greek verb *aisthanomai,*
which means "to sense" or "to know." For the Greeks, sense revealed
knowledge; knowledge was a matter of the sensual. The word *eidenai,*
"to know," is a derivative of *idein,* "to see." One sees first, then one
knows.

In its original sense, aesthetics was not confined to that which was
decorative, pretty, or pleasing, but was used to bespeak all forms, all
that could be perceived. It was not divorced from knowledge but was
the very means through which one learned. It was not separated from
action but was considered an action itself, one of "breathing in."[3]
Through its connection with breath, a metaphor of soul, *aisthesis* was
associated with soul itself.[4]

The modern sense of the word *beauty* was encompassed in the
Greek idea of *kalos. Kalos* was associated with appearance in the sense
of what could be looked at, the sensuous, outer form, that which was
fair and shapely, of fine quality, handsome, and attractive.[5] It referred
to persons, body parts, arms and armor, buildings, and manufactured
articles. The connection of *kalos* to appearance extended to the self-
presentation of persons and gods. It was associated with wealth and
physical well-being. In regard to action, *kalos* was related to sacrifice,
honor, nobility of conduct, justice, honesty, the admirable, the creditable, the straightforward, and "doing right." What we consider as
"quality," was associated by the Greeks with appearance.

*Kalos* connoted that of which the value was apparent, or that which
was desirable for its own sake. It pertained to that wherein the value
did not lie in serving another function but was an end in itself.
According to Hans-Georg Gadamer, *kalos* was opposed to that which
was connected with "use" or that which was in the service of something else.

Hence the idea of the beautiful moves very close to that of the good (*agathon*), insofar as it is something to be chosen for its own sake, as an end that subordinates everything else to it as a means. For what is beautiful is not regarded as a means to something else.[6]

In sum, the notion of *kalos* carried the connotation that appearance was not simply an attribute but an end in and of itself, containing all that was necessary for meaning.

Etymologically, *kalos* is connected to *kaleo*, the act of calling. Plato considered *kalos* to be associated with the action, "to provoke" (*Cratylus*, 416). Calling and provoking suggest the power of appearance itself to move the soul. Because the soul is the "self-mover" (*Phaedrus*, 245 c-d), there must be something of soul in appearance.

The modern counterpart to *kalos* is *beauty*. Beauty comes from the Latin *bellus*, meaning pretty, handsome, charming, or smart. Frequently, it was used ironically to mean fine or excellent. Beauty traditionally conveyed perfection of form and charm of coloring. It was associated with pleasure for the senses and the intellectual faculties through perfection and harmony.[7]

It would seem that the Roman sense of beauty stripped it of the force and polyvalence it held for the Greeks. What started as a notion of perception of forms, the plurality of appearances, and was intricately associated with action, knowledge, and the good, became transformed into a monistic notion—one that lacked necessity and that had to do exclusively with charm and pleasure.

It is this diminished sense of beauty that the modern mind inherits. In modern consciousness, beauty is not an objective force in the world as it was for the Greeks, but an attribute of something that causes pleasure in the subject. In the modern sense, beauty is a subjective phenomenon, lying in the eye of the beholder. To speak of beauty seems effete, ineffectual, soft, and ethereal. We want hard facts, which we locate in mathematics and statistics, to represent the world of truth. Beauty is associated with outer attributes and ornamentation. It is not considered substantial, and, therefore, it is dispensable. Since beauty is not essential, it is not part of the foundation and necessity of our existence but something we locate in the corners and tangential areas of our lives, such as in art objects and nature. Beauty becomes something to be patronized and preserved, but not something to be relied upon or given priority.

Aesthetics, as perception of appearance, and beauty are connected through their association with the Greek notion of *kalos*. In this book I shall try to recover the paradigm of beauty as appearance, one that

imagines the worlds of perception, action, appearance, and truth as one. I will also attempt to show that a paradigm of beauty based on a concept of order is spiritual in origin and leads to methodology that splits appearance from truth and perception from action. Finally, I shall try to show that the former paradigm provides for psychology a particularly appropriate model of inquiry, in that it allows for a dwell-ing of consciousness in the unification of the spiritual and the material.

A psychological understanding of beauty considers it not as an abstraction or a subjective experience, but as a principle of spirit and matter together as revealed in the concrete world. In this sense, beauty is the revealing of the psychological reality inherent in the appearance of things and events. Martin Heidegger wrote, "Our current name for the sight and appearance of something is 'image.' The nature of the image is to let something be seen."[8] Appearance as image, the shining forth of the truth of things, is related to the Greek notion of *aletheia,* the "unconcealedness" of being.

> Truth is the unconcealedness of that which is as something that is. Truth is the truth of Being. When truth sets itself into the work, it appears. Appearance—as this being of truth in the work and as work—is beauty.[9]

Following Heidegger, Gadamer writes, "In regard to beauty, the beau-tiful must always be understood ontologically as an 'image'."[10] In this model of beauty, meaning is regarded as being given in perception, truth lying in the perfection inherent in each particular image.

Beauty can be considered as a way of seeing.[11] Aesthetic or image perception is not just sensate perception, nor fantasy, but a combina-tion of what we usually separate as inner and outer perception. One Greek term for image is *eidos,* "that which is seen," "that which presents itself," or "that which is manifest to seeing." *Eidos* is per-ceived through *phainesthati*—imagination. Aesthetic vision, then, is an imaginative vision that is prior to an inner/outer distinction.

Beauty, as a matter of aesthetic vision, could also be described as the gaze through an "erotic eye."[12] In Greek, the word for "to be with," *sutenai,* also means sexual intercourse. The aesthetic vision ap-prehends truth through connection with the world of appearance, rather than by distancing from appearance via objectification and deriving conclusions through methodology. Understanding through beauty could be considered as the encounter with that which appears. Each apprehension of form would be a coming to know through "being with" the form.

The recovery of beauty entails a translocation of its place from the periphery to the ground of consciousness. Beauty would not be seen as

tangential to the core of experience, located in art, decoration, and ornamentation for the sake of pleasure, or segmented off into nature to be preserved.[13] Rather, beauty would be considered as that which makes everyday consciousness possible. Beauty would then be re-aligned with the Platonic notion that the order of beauty is analogous to the order of being.

Finally, the paradigm of beauty as appearance restores to beauty its grounding in the depths of horror and darkness. I shall not adopt a romantic interpretation of beauty wherein only that which is in align-ment with an underlying, universal order of perfection can be consid-ered as beautiful. In this tradition, Keats wrote:

Some shape of beauty moves away the pall
From our dark spirits.

(Endymion)

Kathleen Raine gives an example of the romantic interpretation of beauty.

Yet, try as we may to come to terms with the ugly and the vulgar, they continue to shock, hurt and jar some intuitive sense of fitness of form and the truth of beauty. . . . the formless and the deformed can only disinte-grate and lacerate, whereas images of order unify and heal. . . . The beau-tiful, then, is the active principle in any work of transforming power, summoning us to self-knowledge of the innate human norm to which we always tend, but from which we always deviate; and the greater the disparity between a sordid actuality, and the perfection of the beautiful, the greater, not the less, is the need for the 'truth' of beauty, to rectify and inform the formless reality—or unreality—of the everyday world.[14]

Here, the power of beauty lies only in its connection to a hidden norm—wholeness, harmony, unity, or perfection.[15] As Raine attests, this is a view that is compatible with a spiritual view of humanity.[16]

In contrast, I am suggesting a vision that would see beauty in deviancy, "sordid actuality," and fragmentation. The gnarled forms in the work of Grünewald and modern sculptors, for example, arrest our attention so that we begin to sense a perfection inherent in frag-mented, as well as ordered, form. With Rilke we would envision beauty as the "beginning of Terror we're still just able to bear,"[17] or with Plotinus be "stricken by a salutary terror" in the sight of beauty,[18] or with Wallace Stevens consider death as the mother of beauty. Like Yeats, we would then be able to see not only the "terrible" in the forms that readily present themselves as beautiful, but the beautiful in the grotesque, deformed, disheveled, skewed, and death-

like forms of life. Beauty's connection with psyche would be in an association with death and darkness, which mythologically are the soul's natural habitats.[19]

I have emphasized the pervasive quality of beauty in the paradigm of beauty as appearance. The idea that there is terror in beauty and horror in forms, however, brings up images at the borderline of this paradigm and notions of the ugly within it. While I have been positing that beauty can be considered as a matter of form or image, differentiated and consistent, shining through the world, Neil Micklem asserts that some images are archetypally unendurable.[20] An example of the archetypally intolerable image in contemporary life would be the atomic bomb. This is an expression of the border of human imagination, yet an image nonetheless, differentiated into details of flashing destruction, and mushrooming devastation, all deepened by mythic backgrounds of divine punishment, stolen fire, and the end of the world.[21]

Micklem points out that the mythic figure of Medusa gives a prototype of the intolerable image. Medusa was once a beautiful woman who slept with Poseidon in a temple to Athene. As punishment, Athene turned her into a winged monster with glaring eyes, huge, tusk-like teeth, protruding tongue, bronze claws, and hair of serpents. In this form, Medusa lived near the edge of the world and turned into stone whoever looked at her directly. Here is an image of beauty turned into terror, existing on the edge of human experience, impossible to behold directly.

Perseus overcame Medusa with the help of Hermes and Athene. Hermes gave him the cap of invisibility and winged sandals for flight. Athene gave him a sword and shield with which to see the monster through her reflection. The myth says that the intolerable image can be survived only through an invisible posture and a reflective vision resulting in an action of stealth. As Micklem says, "Apparently this sort of indirection is a health-giving, life-saving quality that belongs to a vital deviousness of the Gods."[22]

The intolerable image is still an image in its definite form, consistency, and differentiation. Rafael Lopez Pedraza introduces another borderline image that he terms "titanic."[23] The Titans were giants that existed during the second generation of the Greek gods, before the age of Zeus. They were characterized by undifferentiated, massive force, whereas the gods ruled by Zeus were highly differentiated. Titanic phenomena are those of excess, lack of boundary, lack of form, lawlessness, lack of order, and emptiness. Titanic images are images of non-image. The gassing of Jews in mass proportions during World War II (what Arendt referred to as "the banality of evil"),[24] the secretive

administration of capital punishment through lethal injection, commer-
cial television, political newspeak—all these give evidence of an insid-
ious, inhuman lack of imagination in contemporary life, the horror of
an age of "an-esthesia."

Within the paradigm of beauty as the appearance of forms, the idea
of "the ugly" would also need to be delineated. For Plato, ugliness is
that which is "at odds with the divine" (Sym. 206d).[25] Plotinus gives
one of his definitions of ugliness as follows: "We possess beauty when
we are true to our own being; our ugliness is in going over to another
order" (En. V.8.13). For Marsilio Ficino, something is more or less
beautiful to the extent that it agrees with its ideal form or essence:
"Things are judged more or less beautiful according to the proximity of
the first beauty."[26] Ugliness, then, is not that which is asymmetrical,
dark, deviated from a norm, fragmented, or quantitatively lacking in
goodness. Rather, it is that which is out of alignment with the divinity
or truth of its own being. In other words, Plotinus and Ficino would
seem to be postulating a particular perfection, truth, or order for each
individual thing or event. Beauty shines through when the particularity of this order is adhered to. An image is ugly when it is not
well crafted, when it makes an inauthentic appearance, unaligned
with its own unique, intrinsic being.

In relation to psychotherapy, for example, neurosis might be considered as ugliness, not being true to the uniqueness of one's own being.
Following Jung, the aesthetic sense of psychopathology would see
neurosis, not so much from the standpoint of emotional suffering as
such, but from the standpoint of inauthentic suffering displaying itself.
When one is not true to one's unique experience, symptoms present
themselves as a display of that experience. As I will attempt to show in
chapter 8, the aesthetic psychotherapist, by reflecting the image that is
presented, helps to bring about a realignment in the psyche of the
patient.

The method of this work is at once historical and imaginative. I will
present aspects of traditional views of beauty as cornerstones of two
major paradigms of beauty. The figure of Aphrodite introduces the first
paradigm, which holds beauty to be appearance itself. The pillars of
this model lie in the thought of Plato (428 B.C.–348 B.C.), Plotinus
(205 A.D.–270 A.D.) and Ficino (1433 A.D.–1499 A.D.). Plato portrayed the desire for beauty as the central factor in the movement
toward truth. Plotinus, "the philosopher of love and beauty" and the
Roman teacher of Platonism, placed beauty in the center of the universe as the ground of being and provided a sense of the unity of seeing
and doing. Ficino, the Florentine court philosopher, contributed the
image of beauty as the numinosity of light, rhythmically flowing

through the universe and back to God, the source. In presenting this model, I will attempt to show how it both reveals the inherent psychological value of beauty and holds value for psychology as an imaginative discipline of soul.

The second part of the work will focus upon the paradigm of beauty inherited by modern consciousness—that is, beauty as an inner judge-ment. In this paradigm meaning is separated from appearance, thereby diminishing beauty and making the paradigm less useful for a psychol-ogy that finds its home in the unity of the two. I shall introduce this paradigm with a chapter that illustrates a turn away from appearance in paganism, early Christianity, and Protestantism, toward spiritual faith and reason. I shall then connect the spiritual sense of beauty with the concept of proportion and the evolution of proportion into linear perspective. Linear perspective will then be shown to be the founda-tion for the subjectivization of beauty during the Enlightenment.

The paradigm of beauty as an inner experience focuses upon the connection of beauty as a spiritual, conceptual (proportion), meth-odological (linear perspective), and subjective phenomenon. In the tradition of proportion and subjectivism, knowledge is gained through perception that occurs via an organizing system, such as mathematics, or a concept, rather than through the direct perception of appearance. Meaning is separated from perception, and the organizing system, not appearance, becomes the ground of knowledge. Beauty, as the direct, "disinterested" perception of form giving rise to pleasure, and divorced from meaning and action in the world, becomes subordinate to con-cept. I shall suggest that the interiorization of beauty in this paradigm takes place in the service of a need for identification with divinity, control over the physical world, and certainty of consciousness.

Part 3 will attempt to conclude the work by revealing aspects of contemporary psychology—i.e., depth psychology, phenomenological psychology, and psychotherapy—to be the loci for the return of beauty as appearance in contemporary life. In focusing upon the work of Carl Jung in particular, I shall discuss the modern ambivalence toward beauty. Early in his career Jung denigrated aesthetics and upheld a conceptual system of interpretation, while in his more mature writings he equated image with psyche. In approaching psychotherapy, I shall use the models of the *vita contempliva* and the *vita activa* to illustrate how beauty as appearance emerges in the therapeutic situation. Fi-nally, drawing on both Gadamer and Hillman, I shall attempt to envision psychology as an aesthetic way of seeing that brings together the modern splits between spirit and matter, art and science, subject and object.

This book does not approach aesthetics as a discipline of philosophy,

rather it regards aesthetics as a way of being, therefore psychological. It is not a survey of Western thought regarding beauty, but it attempts to see through two major paradigms of beauty to the implications for psychology that underlie each. It is not a call for returning to a consciousness of the past, such as that of the Renaissance or antiquity, but an attempt to both recover beauty as a mode of psychological understanding and to bring psychological understanding to beauty.

In conclusion, beauty is archetypal. All people, across cultures and throughout the ages, have ways of beautifying themselves and their world. Everyone finds beauty in something. No thing or event exists that may not hold beauty. As archetype, beauty is a matter of soul. As a discipline of soul, it is important for psychology to realign itself with beauty. George Russell has made this explicit in his statement, "One of the first symptoms of the loss of the soul is the loss of the sense of beauty."[27] Because beauty is essential to the nature of psyche, it is necessary for psyche's full realization to occur. To recover beauty for the heart of its own being, psychology would concern itself as much with the appearance of things, as with constructs, concepts, and systems. It would look to its constructs, concepts, and systems not so much as tools for the gain of knowledge, but for the aesthetic value inherent in each. For a psychology of aesthetics, the question would be not, "What is the cause?" but rather, "How does it appear?" The aesthetic psychologist would be able to see the value inherent in each symptom, abnormality, grotesquerie, and aberrancy. The therapist, seeing aesthetically, would look for meaning in the detail of the symptom that appears in the moment, rather than to theory, system, or conceptual model. In sum, aesthetic seeing would return ontological value to image and image to psychology, revealing beauty as image to be the psyche's basic ground of data.

# THE SOUL OF BEAUTY

# PART ONE
# BEAUTY AS APPEARANCE

1

# APHRODITE

As an introduction to the paradigm of beauty as appearance, I would like to start with image itself, a personification of beauty as divine in the figure of the Greek goddess Aphrodite. The importance of beauty in the everyday life of the Greeks was reflected in their worship of Aphrodite. For the Greeks, beauty was a power, a force that animated the world, not simply a matter of passing enjoyment. The Greek culture was based on the civilizing influence of beauty, and mythically speaking, the Greeks could be said to have gone to war for the sake of beauty. Homer reflects this Greek attitude in his description of how the old men of Troy, sitting at the Skaian gates, gazed upon Helen above the walls and uttered,

> Surely there is no blame on Trojans and
>     strong-greaved Achians
> If for long time they suffer hardship
>     for a woman like this one!

(Illiad III 156–57)[1]

To recover the psychological value of beauty, we would need to restore the "metaphysical dignity" it held for the Greeks.[2] This would require entering into the world of Aphrodite, the divine personification of beauty.[3]

Although many of the Greek goddesses were described as being beautiful, Aphrodite was considered the essence of beauty. In one of the Homeric hymns, the gods were "amazed by the beauty / Of violet crowned Cythera."[4] Hesiod described her as "who may be called Woman or Eve or Beauty."[5] Walter Otto refers to Aphrodite's beauty as "pure feminine beauty."[6] Paul Friedrich points out that, whereas Homer usually describes beauty by speaking of it indirectly in terms of its effects, the physical details of Aphrodite are described directly.[7] When the Homeric writer wants to praise a woman's beauty most highly, he or she compares her with Aphrodite.

Aphrodite's beauty is that which appears beautiful, not because of conformity to an external norm, but through an unself-conscious,

radiant presence. Morike writes of this beauty, "What is beautiful, appears blissful in itself."[8] The classical valuing of presence is reflected in the Renaissance painting of Botticelli *The Birth of Venus.* Kenneth Clark writes of Botticelli's painting, "It is the strength of Venus that her face reveals no thought beyond the present."[9]

The significance of Aphrodite's presence for psychology is that she does not take us on a hermeneutical movement to a meaning some' where else or to an Archimedean point away from the world in order to understand. With Aphrodite, there is no distanced, analytical insighting, no hidden logocentric source of meaning. The beauty that shows has inherent psychological value. Aphrodite has no referent beyond herself. Her presence is here-and-now. Her meaning lies in form itself.

Radiance or shining is central to Aphrodite's nature. She is called *pasiphaessa* or "far-shining" and is connected with "shining dawn." Aphrodite's radiance is reflected in the word *ekphanestaton,* which means "emergence above the horizon," "showing itself," "bright-shin-ing," "revealing," or "revealing of secret things." Aphrodite's presence can be seen in the German word *Ersheinung* or "appearance."[10] Aph-rodite's shining is the revealing of what is there in the particular luster of each event or moment. When essence is revealed, in whatever form, Aphrodite is present. She tells us that essence lies not in a system of measure or derived meaning, but in the shining through of appearance. All things shine forth their innate nature through her.

Classically, Aphrodite was depicted with a moist or clinging gar-ment, in the act of disrobing, or in the nude—the only goddess to be so portrayed. She is called Aphrodite Morpho, "the shapely" or "she of various shapes." One might say that in the revealing of form lies divinity, or that there is divinity in shape itself. Through Aphrodite, the splendor of beauty finds its way in all forms; her beauty is what makes the world perceptible. She grounds the sensate particularity of each event in the world. James Hillman remarks that, without Aphro-dite, the particularity of the world becomes just atomic particles and energy.[11]

Aphrodite is the only goddess to reveal herself naked to mortal eyes without punishment. She makes love with the mortal Anchises, who, upon waking from postcoital sleep, finds that he has been with a goddess and fears punishment. Aphrodite soothes him thusly:

Noble Anchises, most glorious of mortal mankind,
Be of good courage and fear not too much in your heart.
You will suffer no evil from me or the other blessed immortals,
For you are dear to the gods.[12]

Through Aphrodite, human vision of the divine in sensuous form is "dear," with no need for guilt, punishment, or self-consciousness, just as in the *Phaedrus* (250d) where beauty is depicted by Plato as the only form accessible to human vision. Henri Corbin asserts that beauty is the "supreme theophany of divine self-revelation."[13] Aphrodite, then, gives divinity or psychological value to display, exhibition, and presentation of self.[14]

The Greeks celebrated physical passion and gave it religious status. Temples to Aphrodite provided facilities for couples to have intercourse in celebration of fertility. In describing the sculpture known as *Cnidian Aphrodite* by Praxitales, Kenneth Clark states:

> Perhaps no religion ever again incorporated physical passion so calmly, so sweetly and so naturally that all who saw her felt that the instincts they shared with beasts, they also shared with the gods. It was a triumph for beauty.[15]

With the intertwining of passion and religion, the clothed with the unclothed, Aphrodite brings together matter and spirit.

The Greeks are saying that when we see sensuously, with a vision that "joins with" in erotic connection, we see through the eyes of Aphrodite. When carnal embrace is visionary, it is the embrace of Aphrodite, sensualizing the mind. The gaze of sensualized consciousness neither penetrates to a "source of truth," nor does it transcend appearance, ascending to an essence beyond. Instead, it engages in foreplay with the surface of appearance, uniting with that which appears on its own ground of being, and allowing for the emergence of perfection in the particular appearance of each strange form.

Alphonso Lingis takes his readers to the ancient Hindu temple of Khajuraho in India for a depiction of erotic seeing.

> What seems to be a universal combination of carnal positions is brought to the same explicitness and precision. Autoerotic stimulation, dual and multiple cunnilinctio, penilinctio, copulation, homosexual and bestial intercourse circulate about the temple walls, without primacy of place or of artistry given to any figure. . . . Here one neither descends when one makes love with animals and trees, nor ascends, when one makes love with the moon, the rivers, the stars; one travels aimlessly or circularly about a universe eroticized.[16]

Here, the 8.4 million forms of animal positions that are the foundation for the 8.4 million *asanas* of Patanjali's classical *hatha yoga* are all taken as human possibilities. Here, the human body not only makes contact with every other organic form, but each separate and unique form of

the individual body has relationship with each unique form of every other body. The dissymmetry of sexes is not a practice of power or ascendance. Men bearing vulvas and women bearing penile erections alternate and reciprocate in initiation and reception. Here, the gaze does not ascend nor descend, penetrate nor detach; it circulates aimlessly, drifting, holding the reverberations between forms. In short, what is revealed at Khajuraho through the depiction of human bodies in supple, erotic connection with the universe is a bodily way of seeing, being as seeing, seeing as embodied, seeing/being/body—all one.

Aphrodite's love and care of mortals was reflected in the quality of her beauty that the Greeks called *charis*, or grace. In grace, there is a rhythm of giving, receiving, and returning with gratitude. The self-enclosed rhythm of grace is projected imagistically in the classical depiction of the Graces, the attendants of Aphrodite, with their arms encircling each other. Grace lies in the self-contained, to-and-fro flowing of Aphrodite's beauty. In this sense, Walter Otto describes her beauty as "loveliness which is at the same time a receptivity and an echo."[17] Kenneth Clark notes the grace of Aphrodite in his description of Botticelli's *Birth of Venus*.

> Her differences from antique form are not physiological but rhythmic and structural. . . . She is not standing, but floating. This is the rhythm of the whole picture. . . . Every movement is related to every other by a line of unbroken grace.[18]

As Aphrodite was the essence of beauty, so also was her beauty intrinsically golden. Her beauty was the beauty of pure, luminous, incorruptible substance associated with gold and with the sun. Pindar wrote, "but gold, like a gleaming fire / by night outshines all pride of wealth beside."[19] Aphrodite was called "Golden Aphrodite," and this adjective was used for her alone. The Greeks considered her to have "joy-creating-sun-like-magic," and associated her with warmth, perfection, and radiance.[20] Through Aphrodite they could take delight in the "joy of image."[21] Aphrodite's consciousness is earthly in feeling and yet bright and lucid in its spirit, earth and heaven united and refined to the highest purity.

The gold of Aphrodite refers both to her spiritually golden qualities and to material gold, her jewelry. Gold as jewelry bespeaks the power of appearance to attract from a distance. The second Homeric hymn to Aphrodite describes her adornment by the Hours.

[T]he gold filleted Hours
Welcomed her gladly and clothed her in ambrosial garments

And on her immortal head set a chaplet of richly wrought gold.
Flowerlike earrings formed of fine brass and rare gold
They fastened them in Aphrodite's pierced ear lobes,
And around her delicate throat and silvery breasts
Hung necklaces inlaid with gold.[22]

Ginette Paris sees the sexuality of women in the radiance of gold as jewelry.[23] In Aphrodite, then, the "sacred" and the "profane" connotations of gold come together. She makes radiance sexual and sex radiant.

The word *cosmetics* is related to the Greek *kosmos,* which originally referred to the right placing of the multiple things of the world. James Hillman notes that *kosmos* also implied aesthetic qualities such as becoming, decent, honorable, and creditable.[24] *Kosmos* was used especially in regard to women's embellishments. The art of adornment with cosmetics and jewelry is a reflection of the right placing of things in the universe. If beauty is seen as the face of things as they are, then making up the face is an honoring of the cosmic face of things.

In addition to her delight in gold jewelry, Aphrodite takes pleasure in all the ornamentations and decorations of love, such as perfume and flowers. What the modern mind thinks of as mere externals or artifice are essential for Aphrodite. When she was in love with Anchises,

She hastened to Cyprus and entered her sweet-smelling temple
In Paphos, where lay her sacred precinct and altar,
And shut behind her the gleaming doors of the shrine.
There the Graces bathed and annointed her, smoothing on ambrosial
    ungents such as perfume of the gods everlasting and
Divinely fragrant oils of the goddess' own.
Then Aphrodite, lover of smiles, clothed in all her fine raiment,
Gold-adorned, flew to Troy, forsaking sweet-scented Cyprus.[25]

As divinity of perfumes, oils, scents, jewelry, and flowers, Aphrodite teaches us that for love to be of the soul, appearance must be attended to in careful detail. For Aphrodite, "putting on the face" is as important as taking off the clothes.

The beauty of Aphrodite is not all lightness and harmony. Aphrodite was born from a monstrous element, the severed genitals of Uranus and the chaos of the primeval waters. According to Hesiod, she bore Terror and Fear, Deimos and Phobus, as her children. She was married to Hephaistos, the ugly, crippled god who worked in the underground. She had the surnames of Melainis, "the black one," and Skotia, "the dark one." At Delphi there was worship of Aphrodite of the Grave, and she was known as the "Grave Robber," "Aphrodite of

Darkness," and "Black Aphrodite." Her image was found on tombs, a goddess of death represented in frozen slumber.

Aphrodite's connection with ugliness and terror reminds one that even the horrid, dark, and grotesque forms have their own beauty.[26] Her dark side can be seen in her mourning the loss of her lover, Adonis, or in her horrible revenges on those who defied her: Hippolytus, the daughters of Tyndareus—Timandra, Helen, and Clytemnestra, who were unfaithful to their husbands with drastic consequences—Pasiphae, who was brought to love a bull, and the Lemnian women, who were given a repellent odor. Claire Lejeune writes:

> This Beauty is sovereign, because it is unforeseeable and inescapable. Against its possible victory, our defeat, we arm ourselves; we turn from terror to terrorism. The ultimate object of human fear is Beauty; nothing is more disarming, more ravishing, than its eruption in our lives. Beauty alone brings us to our knees without abasement, washes away all humiliation, heals us of all rancor, and reconciles us with the universe.[27]

Aphrodite, both radiant and associated with death, gives form to the totality of soul.

In Plotinus's interpretation of Plato, Aphrodite is Soul itself (*En.* III.5.5) Aphrodite's connection with soul can also be seen in the tale of Eros and Psyche. In this tale, Psyche appears as a mortal who is so beautiful she is worshipped on earth in the place of Aphrodite. In other words, Psyche is Venus incarnate. As the story goes, Eros falls in love with Psyche, desire joining with soul. As punishment, Psyche is given a series of tasks by Aphrodite. Here, soul is being worked upon by beauty. From this story, James Hillman points out that we know soul first through her visible, sensate beauty and later through her associations to aspects usually deemed psychological—tasks, sufferings, and being lost.[28] Soul, then, is the life of aesthetic responses.

Aphrodite is the goddess of phenomenological psychology, reminding us of the intentionality of consciousness toward something, as well as the divinity of imaginal psychology, which makes image its ground. Knowledge through Aphrodite's vision, reveals itself via a sensuous view of the world. In contrast to the Apollonian vision, distant and objective, her seeing conjoins with what is there. It is a view of simultaneous giving and taking, being affected by, while affecting. Aphrodite's knowing is one of sensuous delight, an *episteme* of eros.

In approaching Aphrodite psychologically, one would say that through Aphrodite, all appearance is golden, luminous, and radiant. Aphrodite does not refer us, in an interpretive move, to find meaning in an abstract logocentric source—i.e., the latent dream of psycho-

analysis or the self of Jungian psychology. What is necessary is already there. For Aphrodite, every small, sensuous detail of every form is important, the askew as well as the symmetrical. Every slip, symptom, aberrancy, depression, fragment, and failure has a beauty or value of its own. Through Aphrodite, all ornamentation and surface detail is taken as being essence, the depth lying in the surface. Through Aphrodite's eye, meaning lies in appearance itself. She sees reality in appearance and sees in appearance the perfection inherent in each particular form.

2
# BEAUTY AS LIGHT

In this chapter I shall attempt to provide the foundation for a paradigm of beauty as appearance, a paradigm that I shall suggest holds inherent value for psychology. The paradigm, as outlined in the introduction, might be summarized as follows: The aesthetic eye perceives appearance in its particular presenting form. In the perceiving, an image is created, and in the image lies meaning. The power that allows for this process, beauty, is imagined as light—light that allows for the particularity of each thing and event to display its own perfection. At the same time the power of beauty allows for the unity of all being and, as such, is the ground for all experience.

From Aphrodite, one learns that soul is manifested in the appearance of form, bringing together the visible and the invisible. I suggest that this understanding of beauty, "a thing of Matter and . . . Celestial" in Plotinus's words (*En.* III.5.9), which joins matter and spirit, lends itself to a psychological understanding of phenomena. In this paradigm, all appearance is considered psychological, wherever it occurs, and psychology is evoked wherever there is appearance.[1] At the same time, the paradigm integrates the notions of seeing, doing, and knowing through its sense of perception as, at once, creating and knowing. With the paradigm of beauty as appearance, all action in and knowledge of the world is rooted in vision. Finally, within the paradigm of beauty as appearance, appearance and being coincide, making being itself a "matter" of interest for psychology.

I would like to proceed by exploring the different aspects of the paradigm of beauty as appearance as it emerged in the Neoplatonic tradition. This tradition, with its predominant interest in the nature of soul (psyche), offers a particularly relevant model for "psychology" as a study (*logie*) of soul. I have differentiated the pertinent aspects of the Neoplatonic tradition as follows: (1) order, (2) mediation, (3) love, (4) perception, (5) knowledge, (6) light, and (7) unity.

## BEAUTY AND ORDER

The Neoplatonic universe is one of hierarchical ordering in which the multiplicity of existence springs from the unity of the divine source. Hierarchy gives value. In the *Phaedrus* (249e), Plato has Socra-tes describe the divine realm of Forms, *logos,* or "true being" as being separate from the world of matter.[2] In the *Symposium* (211e), Diotima describes in detail the movement of the earthly soul toward these forms as "ever mounting the heavenly ladder" toward divine beauty. For Plotinus, the universe consists of a hierarchical order of levels, each of which is made from a prior realm, extending from the source of being. The order of priority starts with the One, the unity of which is superior to all distinctions and extends through the divine realms of the eternal Forms and the World Soul to the sensate world. In Ficino's image of the universe, a hierarchy of being exists extending from the unity of God, through mind (the multiplicity of ideas,) soul (the incorruptible realm of forms,) and nature, to the world of matter. For Ficino, the Platonic notion of transcendence, Aristotelian categories, and the Christian God are all combined.

In the Plotinian view, the universe, although hierarchical, is ani-mated and connected by the principle of beauty. Beauty as principle, streaming through the prior levels, endows each thing and event with its own particular beauty. It is the realm of Soul, *immediate* to the sensate world that gives matter its shape.

> The beauty in things of a lower order—actions and pursuits for instance—comes by operation of the shaping Soul which is also the author of the beauty found in the world of sense. (*En.* I.6.6)

Things or patterns have their beauty through their connection with a higher beauty, but the creating force is close at hand. In turn, the power of the principle of beauty to bestow the quality of beauty onto the material world comes through its emanation from the divine. Something is beautiful to its degree of alignment with ultimate beauty. Sensible or worldly beauty, then, is a reflection of divine or supreme beauty. Plotinus writes, "This . . . is how the material thing becomes beautiful—by communicating in the thought that flows from the Divine (*En.* I.6.2)." Here the emphasis is less on vertical separation and more on universal interconnection.

For Ficino, God is the center of a hierarchical universe that extends outward. The four subsequent realms are mind (*nous*—multiplicity of ideas, intelligible, incorruptible), soul (incorruptible, self-moving, acausal realm of forms), nature (terrestrial world, movable in another), and matter (formless and lifeless, movable by another). God's radiance

pours out as if overflowing from a fountain in overabundance and emanates to all parts of the universe. Each concentric circle surrounding the center creates the subsequent outer circle under the influence of the divine source. Hence, each circle is contained *a priori* in the subsequent inner circle. The closer each circle is to the center, the purer and more complete is its nature, and the higher it stands in the cosmic hierarchy. Each realm of the cosmology desires both to (1) ascend to the next higher level, its place of origin, and ultimately to its source of being, the center of the universe, *and* (2) descend through procreation to the next realm nearest the material. Again, the emphasis is on the connection, not the distance, between matter and spirit, the seen and the unseen.

In developing a paradigm of beauty as appearance, then, the ordered sense of the Neoplatonic universe is relevant for its vision of the interaction between the different realms through the dynamics of beauty. In this sense, the Renaissance universe is not a symmetrical, logocentric entity. Its equality is that of a circle "whose circumference is nowhere and the center everywhere," to use Nicholas of Cusa's famous phrase.[3] Ficino explains, "And the nature of the center is such that, although it is single, indivisible and motionless, it is nevertheless found . . . everywhere."[4]

For the purposes of the paradigm of beauty as appearance, the reading that A. Hilary Armstrong gives to the Platonic and Neoplatonic order is quite helpful. Armstrong reminds readers that Platonism was formulated in an atmosphere still influenced by the Homeric sense of divinity as interacting with the earthly.

> This very simple fact that the context of Platonism was the old Hellenistic piety needs to be continually remembered. The Platonists lived among the shrines and images of the older world.[5]

Central to the Homeric notion of divine beauties was the sense that they interacted with earthly beauties. Armstrong describes the idea that the beauties of earth and of the gods can be experienced together.

> Earthly beauties stimulate and provide expression for awareness of divine presence, and in turn, the sense of divine presence enhances earthly beauties.[6]

In other words, the beauties of the earth were experienced as such because there was something divine in them. Armstrong continues:

> How, then, can we speak of a divine enhancement of earthly beauty when all earthly beauty is divine? In the Greek, as in all archaic cultures, there is

an intense awareness of the *poikilia* of the one divine world, or the continual variations in kind and degree of the divine manifestations in its beauty.[7]

In the Homeric tradition, then, divine beauty was experienced on earth in a multiplicity of ways—in theophanies, special moments, signs and places. Armstrong writes, "Wild and tame, mad and sane, dark and light: in all these the divine is present, and where it is present there is an intensified beauty."[8]

The major transition from Homeric to Platonic consciousness of beauty was that the latter experienced the divine as trancendent, therefore inaccessible to mortal perception; this transcendent consciousness was imagined in the form of cosmic hierarchy. Armstrong, however, is careful to point out that the separation of material from spiritual is not a spatial separateness of above and below. Plato's Forms, by definition are incorporeal, hence not in space and cannot be considered in relation to the material world with spatial concepts such as *beyond* or *above*.

Armstrong asserts that the emphasis on the spatial transcendence of divinity is due to the influence of "cosmic piety," one aspect of Greek consciousness that originated at the time of Plato and extended into the Gnostic and early Christian worlds. This notion is based upon a view in which the world is small, low, cold, dark, damp, passive, female, and impure, in contrast to the hot, bright, dry, active, male purity of the fire in the heavens. Plato has Socrates say in the *Philebus* (29c) for example,

> And isn't the fire that belongs to ourselves small in quantity and weak and inconsiderable, whereas the fire in the universe is wonderful in respect of its mass, its beauty, and all the powers that belong to fire?[9]

The attitude of cosmic piety sees the world's beauties as being degraded, dimmed, and spoiled, and its delights as transitory and corrupting. Priority is placed on the heavens and the ascent to them. Humans need salvation or escape, and this can only come about by lifting the gaze to the fires of the heavenly world. Armstrong notes that this influence in the Greek tradition led to a despising of the beauties of the earth and established the heavens "beyond" as the place of true, divine beauty. This diminished sense of earthly beauty is the foundation for a definition of beauty based upon mathematical structures of symmetry and proportion. Beauty on earth becomes that which imitates the ideal in its perfect order.

In addition to seeing the influence of "cosmic piety" in Plato, however, Armstrong detects a notion of beauty that tends toward the

Homeric vision of beauty. In arguing for a reading that sees the
presence of the divine in the earthly, Armstrong emphasizes such
Platonic ideas as the particularity of earthly beauty as the starting
point of the ascent toward truth, the enhancement of earthly beauty
by the universal, the importance of horizontal as well as vertical
expansion, and the possibility of descent as well as ascent on Diotima's
ladder.

A close look at Diotima's description of the movement of the soul
toward beauty bears out Armstrong's reading. The soul to be initiated
into the mysteries of love and beauty is drawn first toward the beauties
of the physical body. This move toward body affirms the corporeal
origins of our vision. The soul realizes that the beauty of one body is
related to the beauty of any other. It becomes the lover of every "lovely
body" or one might say, "a lover of the loveliness in every body." To
see the truth of the various forms of corporeal beauty in this way is to
see *noetic* beauty, the beauty of *nous* or wisdom.

Although Diotima characterizes the progressive movement of the
soul as "ever mounting the heavenly ladder (*Sym.* 211)," her actual
description portrays both vertical and horizontal movement. In fact,
she speaks of the erotic gaze as "scanning beauty's wide horizon" (*Sym.*
210 d). It would seem that, as Armstrong asserts, Diotima is describing
the ability to see beauty in an ever-widening way, taking in the here-
and-now in an ever more complete manner, so that the particular
beauty of each thing and event can be apprehended. Beauty is not
beyond so much as "right there" for the loving eye to embrace.

The argument for a Neoplatonic foundation honoring earthly
beauty runs into a particular problem in Plotinus's disparaging attitude
toward bodily being and his emphasis on mystical union with the
One.[10] Porphyry wrote that his teacher Plotinus "seemed ashamed of
being in his body," and refused to sit for a portrait.[11] In his treatise
"On Beauty" Plotinus asserts that for a vision of "loftier beauties"
(*En.* I.6.4) consciousness must leave the sensual world. This is
achieved by one who will "withdraw into himself, foregoing all that is
known by the eyes, turning away forever from the material beauty that
once made his joy" (*En.* I.6.8). Such a one must "close the eyes and call
instead upon another vision which is to be waked within" (*En.* I.6.8).
In fact, here Plotinus defines the ugly as that which is embodied. "So,
we may justly say, a Soul becomes ugly—by something foisted upon it,
by sinking itself into the alien, by a fall, a descent into body, into
Matter" (*En.* I.6.5).

> What else is *Sophrosyny*, rightly so-called, but to take no part in the
> pleasures of the body, to break away from them as unclean and unworthy
> of the clean? So too, Courage is but being fearless of the death which is but

the parting of the Soul from the body, an event which no one can dread whose delight is to be his unmingled self. (*En.* I.6.6)

Plotinus's emphasis upon disembodiment and mystical union can be viewed as one side of his thought, a side that stands in reaction to materialism and literalism. Following Armstrong, however, there is another side of Plotinus wherein the emphasis is placed upon the proximity of heavenly beauty to earthly beauty. It is this reading of Plotinus that I feel lends itself more to a psychological sense of beauty, bringing the spiritual and the material closer together. Armstrong stresses that in Plotinus, both the divine Forms and the material world are nourished by the beauty of the One, thus giving a unity to divine and material being. The Forms and the earthly beauties are beautiful because of the light that radiates from the One and plays upon them. Secondly, the primary quality of the One as the infinite source of radiance is the good, the warmth of generosity that flows to all beings, material and spiritual. Finally, Armstrong notes that it is soul, not the Forms, that creates and governs the material world. The archetype is *immediately* present to the image it forms.

It is Soul, not Intellect in Plotinus which forms, governs and animates the material cosmos, imparting to it its proper degree of diversity: but this does not make the intelligible cosmos more remote from the sense world. Hier-archical superiority in the Neoplatonists does not mean greater re-moteness.[12]

I suggest that Plotinus's sense of the vision of the beautiful as a leaving of the body is not so much a mystical, as it is a contemplative vision that sees through the literal. This is a recognition that the beauties of the divine and of the earth are not entirely separate. Contemplation undermines a dualistic subject and object separation—"see no longer in that mode of separation" (*En.* V.8.10)—and allows for "inner" and "outer" to play off of each other. The beauty of what is, is "in here" and "out there" at one and the same time. Plotinus writes, "When, from that outward form, the lover elaborates within himself in his own partless soul an immaterial image, then it is that love is born" (*En.* V.7.33). Plotinus is moving not only from outer to inner, but from particular to universal, from the literal to the image located between the physical and the ideal. He is "seeing through" the ontological hierarchy, seeing through the literal to the life of each thing and event in its appearance.

Armstrong asserts that Plotinus thus moves Platonism away from a static sense of the Forms, enabling an appreciation of the divine pres-ence in the beauties of the earth.

Formal perfection in the full sense of the finite perfection of the World of Forms which contains all real being is not enough. It needs, and of course eternally receives a light and life from the Form-less which alone is what the soul, driven on by the eros which is given by that Good, truly seeks.[13]

According to Armstrong, Plotinus provides the opportunity "for valuing the imperfect and changing, but lovely and endlessly various beauties of this earth of ours."[14] In this reading, earth matters because it participates in the beauty of the divine. "What is this that gives grace to the corporeal?" Plotinus asks. "The participation in beauty" (*En.* V.9.2)—the participation of all imperfect, finite things in the perfection of the infinite is what makes the perception of the universe possible. What was for Homeric man, Aphrodite shining through the things of the world to make them perceptible, is for Plotinus, the principle of beauty.

In concluding, Armstrong suggests that the sense of the material realm as image manifesting divine archetype on the physical level is essential for the Platonic awareness of divine presence in and enhancement of the physical world. However, throughout the Platonic tradition there is an ambiguity regarding the valuing of the image. One emphasis is on the isolation of the image from the archetype and on the inferiority of the former. The other emphasis is upon the excellence of the image on its proper level, "this perceptible god, image of the intelligible, greatest and best, most beautiful and most perfect," as Armstrong translates Plato's last sentence of the *Timaeus.*[15] It is the ground of implications underlying this latter attitude that I wish to explore in forming a psychological paradigm of beauty.

The argument for the de-stratified nature of Neoplatonic order has been prolonged because it serves the paradigm of beauty as appearance and enhances psychology. It allows for a more comprehensive sense of beauty than a spiritualized notion, which emphasizes the remoteness of the divine and utilizes systems or methods that imitate the idea. In reference to psychology this would mean relativizing the mode that employs methodology (experimental method and statistical analysis) in order to approximate a distant "truth" (scientific reliability and validity). In terms of depth psychology, this would mean de-emphasizing systems of interpretation in terms of concepts (Freudian structural theory or Jungian topology, theory of oppositions and compensation, and the self concept) in favor of focusing on the actual experience of the patient. The sense of beauty that sees the divine in the earthly would allow for beauty to be manifested in each earthly form, the "dark other" of the Platonic vision. Psychology would see truth in the experience of events and the appearance of phenomena. Appearance

would matter, not as simply sensate perception, but as the embodiment of mind, spirit, or ideal. Following Heraclitus, the Plato of the *Symposium,* and Ficino, the aesthetic vision of appearance would deepen, widen, and decentralize psychological vision to enable imaginal seeing or what James Hillman calls "seeing through" phenomena to the particular truth of their being.

## BEAUTY AS MEDIATOR

In the Neoplatonic cosmos, beauty is the mediator between the separate realms. For Plato, of all the Forms, only beauty is accessible to human perception. "For beauty alone, this has been ordained to be most manifest to sense and most lovely of them all (*Phae.* 250 d).[16] This sense of beauty as mediator is reminiscent of Aphrodite as the sole goddess to reveal herself to mortal eyes.

The idea of beauty as mediator is crucial for the paradigm of beauty as appearance, because it makes beauty the ground of consciousness. Things are because they are beautiful. Beauty is what animates the world, revealing a spark of divinity or perfection in every thing or event that makes its appearance. As Hillman summarizes, beauty is the "shining forth of the hidden noumenal Gods and imperceptible virtues."[17]

Stanley Rosen sees in Plato the love of beauty as the bridge between everyday life and the realm of divine ideas.[18] It is a bridge that carries two paths. The divine needs the corporeal to achieve completeness in visibility, and humanity can find totality only in the vision of the divine achieved through the desire for beauty. Suspended between bodily death and the perfection of soul in the realm of ideas, human beings have only the enduring power of beauty as guide and perpetuator of existence. The divine has only beauty as its means of manifesting itself as an enduring presence in the daily world. Here, the power of the beautiful is immediately perceptible in a way the power of the true and good is not.

Likewise, for Plotinus, the two worlds of the universal and the particular, the divine and the corporeal, cannot exist without the other. The divine needs the corporeal through which to manifest itself. The corporeal needs the divine as its source and light. "Matter is needed to the producing" (*En.* V.7.33). Plotinus asserted, "By what image can we represent it [Form]? We have nowhere to go but to what is less" (*En.* V.8.3). Through the interaction of the two differentiated realms, the spiritual and the material, the universe is paradoxically a unity and a plurality, the one and the many at once. "The duality, thus

is a unity" (*En.* III.8.8). Things have, at once, a universal and an individual aspect. The universal aspect is necessary for the animation of the particular. The individual aspect is necessary in order for the particular to be perceived as such, i.e., for consciousness of the thing to occur. It is beauty that provides the possibility for this simultaneous display and perception.

Nowhere is the coparticipation of the divine and material realms more evident than in the Renaissance sense of man's relation to God. The medieval mode of understanding the world was through transcen-dence from the things of earth to the wonders of heavenly life. The world was made of objects animated and moved by God. The universe was a transcendental hierarchy leading to divinity, everything in the universe pointing to God. By contrast, the mark of Renaissance con-sciousness was that understanding was achieved through the natural world.

The Renaissance mind understood the intelligible to be revealed through the sensible. Nicholas of Cusa, for example, thought that divine truth of the One presented itself in the "other" and simulta-neously the "other" pointed to essential divine unity.[19] Each world, although separate from the other, participates with the other. Cusa taught that the divine One could only be seen in the worldly other. He did not recognize any notions of hierarchical distance between the sensible and the supersensible. Everything is equally far and near from the original source of being. Everything is equally "immediate to God."[20] In everything there is a "trace of God."[21] The difference we perceive in things is a matter of proportion in the mixture of basic elements that are disseminated throughout the world. The par-ticularity of each thing is not a limitation but, in fact, a value. It is only through the particular that the divine "beyond being" can be grasped.[22]

In the development of his doctrine, Cusa emphasized the revelation of God in the particularity of each thing. God's interpenetration into the earthly world is a revealing of his "face." The individual can see himself only in God, just as he can see God only in himself.

Your true face is free of all limitations. It is neither of this size, nor of this shape, neither spatial nor temporal, for it is itself the absolute form, the face of faces. And when I consider how this face is the truth and the most adequate measure of all faces, I am astounded. For this face, that is the truth of all faces, is not this or that large, has no "more" or "less," nor is it like any other; as the absolute, it transcends all measure. So I see, oh Lord, that your face precedes every visible face, that is the truth and the model of all faces. Therefore, any face that looks into yours sees nothing different from itself, because it sees its own truth.[23]

When we "face" the world itself, without tools for understanding, or address the bare face of the world, the world reveals its truth to us.

In the Renaissance Neoplatonic model, the material looks to the spiritual for life, while the spiritual desires the material for the sake of its revealing. The result is a circuit of desire and care extending from God through the levels of being to matter and then returning to God in gratitude. Man's striving toward God in love is reciprocated by God's reaching toward man in care and concern. The intelligible seeks the sensible, the sensible strives for the infinite. Each realm creates and cares for its inferiors. Each life impulse moves out from its source through the act of creation. This intention is reciprocated by a desire for a return to the source. In this dual movement, the opposition between the intelligible and the sensible is unified. Again, Aphrodite is evoked with her gift of giving and receiving. The continuous stream of love emanating from God to earth and returning to God in gratitude is the dynamic of grace.

The Renaissance Neoplatonic notion of transcendence emphasizes relationship rather than a leaving of one realm for another. Cusa and Ficino envisioned each element of the universe as pointing to or symbolizing another that was higher on the scale. Hence, the meta-physics of symbolization and the language of metaphor were vital to them. The symbol connected the general and universal to the par-ticular and to the immediate sensible. The tangible or finite symbolized that which was infinite. Neoplatonic symbolization, however, was not simply a dualistic system of referral. That which was higher in the hierarchy could not exist without being manifest in the lower. Cusa said, "The separation (between the sensible and the ideal) guarantees the possibility of true participation of the sensible in the ideal."[24] The higher can only become manifest, only be grasped through its actu-alization in the lower, guaranteeing the lower participation in the divine, and insuring it a vital place in the cosmic hierarchy. Through the symbol, one sees the signified in the signifier, or the "One in the other," in Cusa's words. Rather than being a system of lifeless sign referring to vital source, symbolization embodies paradoxical coexis-tence. Hence, the Renaissance Neoplatonic view of beauty as mediator helps psychology by moving away from an interpretive mode and, instead, by seeing depth *in* the surface, soul *in* the world, mind *in* the flesh.

## LOVE

In the Neoplatonic universe, harmony exists because of the rela-tionship of attraction and care engendered by *love* among the disparate

parts, and it is beauty that attracts love. All love regards beauty as its end and comes to rest in beauty. In the *Phaedrus,* Socrates refers to beauty as the object of love.

> When irrational desire, pursuing the enjoyment of beauty, has gained the mastery over judgement that prompts to right conduct, and has acquired from other desires, akin to it, fresh strength to strain toward bodily beauty, that very strength provides it with its name—it is the strong passion called love. (*Phae.* 238 c)
>
> And when he that loves beauty is touched by such madness, he is called a lover. Such a one, as soon as he beholds the beauty of this world, is reminded of true beauty. (*Phae.* 249 d)

Likewise, for Plotinus, those who are attuned to beauty are, in fact, lovers.

> This is the spirit that Beauty must ever induce, wonderment and a delicious trouble, longing and love and a trembling that is all delight. (*En.* I.6.4)
>
> What is this Dionysiac exultation that thrills through your being, this straightening upwards of all your soul? (*En.* I.6.5)
>
> The Beauty supreme, the absolute and the primal, fashions its lovers to Beauty and makes them also worthy of Love. (*En.* I.6.7)

Beauty moves the soul, and the soul's attitude toward beauty is one of passion, as described by Plato. He distinguishes between the movement toward beauty of the heavenly and of the earthly soul in love.[25] When the heavenly soul,

> fresh from the mystery (of true beauty, beholds a) bodily form that truly expresses beauty . . . she throbs with ferment in every part . . . feels a ferment and painful irritation . . . [and] admits a flood of particles streaming therefrom—that is why we speak of a "flood of passion"—whereby she is warmed and fostered. (*Phae.* 251 a–c)

The earthly soul is divided into three parts, the charioteer and two steeds.[26] One horse is white, upright, a lover of glory, with temperance and modesty—the reasoned pursuer of beauty. The other horse is black, the image of willful, lustful desire,

> crooked of frame, a massive jumble of a creature with thick short neck, snub nose, black skin, and gray eyes, hot-blooded, consorting with wantoness and vainglory, shaggy of ear, deaf and hard to control. (*Phae.* 253 e)

The chairoteer does not need to concern himself with the white horse

who is self-controlled; but with the black "he jerks back the bit in the mouth . . . bespatters his railing tongue and his jaws with blood, and forcing him down on legs and haunches delivers him over to anguish" (*Phae.* 254e). In this Homeric description, one can see the earthly soul making its way toward beauty, lurching and jarring in a movement beset with pain and blood.

For Plotinus as well, the passion of erotic perception is not pleasing but a source of pain, "the keener wound" (*En.* I.6.5). "Beauty for the knowing and awakened sets up pain and urge to pursue . . . in pain of love towards beauty" (*En.* V.5.2., V.9.2). How different the sense of aesthetic perception as passionate, painful desire is from the subjec- tivist paradigm where aesthetic perception is "disinterested" and ac- companied only by the feeling of pleasure.

Ficino's universe is animated by love. All movement of the soul comes from love, and love regards beauty as its end. There are two kinds of love—heavenly and earthly or vulgar.[27] These two loves can be distinguished by the desire to return to origins on the one hand, and the desire to procreate on the other. The desire to return to the source by striving toward the spiritual or universal realm is heavenly love, the desire for spiritual renewal. Vulgar love is the desire to procreate through a striving toward the material. In Ficino's words, "It is the desire for procreation with a beautiful object in order to make eternal life available to mortal things."[28]

Following Plato, Ficino personifies the two loves in two forms of Venus—Celestial Venus who dwells in the highest zone of the uni- verse, the cosmic mind, and Venus Vulgaris who dwells between the cosmic mind and the sublunary world.

> Therefore, let there be two Venuses in the World Soul, the first heavenly and the second vulgar. Let both have a love: the heavenly for contemplat- ing divine Beauty, the vulgar for procreating the same in the Matter of the World. . . . The heavenly Venus strives, through its intelligence, to re- produce in itself as exactly as possible the beauty of the higher things; the vulgar Venus strives, through the fertility of its divine seeds, to reproduce in the Matter of the World the beauty which is divinely conceived within itself.[29]

In sum, each realm of the hierarchy looks to the prior realm as its source for renewal while caring for the subsequent realm as its crea- tion.

Finally, for Ficino, beauty calls or "provokes" the soul to God.[30] It is the grace of the cosmos that draws the soul to desire its own perfection and so turn back in love to God who can supply its need. Beauty, as the "splendor and grace" of God's face, makes its pleasing to

the soul.[31] "God draws the desire of the mind to Himself by filling it with beauty, and by drawing desire to himself he fulfills it."[32] Love for God is a superior love in that as beauty attracts the soul to God, so the soul becomes beautiful itself.

Love is important for a psychological sense of beauty and for an aesthetic sense of psychology because it provides for a dynamism of soul. Soul, as "self-mover" (*Phae.* 245 c–d) is moved by love. The movement of soul is both regressive—causal oriented, inclined toward origins (psychoanalytic drive theory, developmental theory, behaviorism)—and progressive—drawn toward the goal (humanistic self-actualization, Jungian individuation). Through eros the life of soul becomes one of teleology as well as causality, purpose as well as instinct. The psychotherapeutic question becomes as much, "What is drawing the soul in this direction?" as "What is causing this to occur?"

Through love, understanding becomes "being with" and "caring for" image, rather than distancing from the object for the sake of control and certainty. The aesthetic vision sees appearance as much as possible within the context of its presentation. The view is not from the bird's eye of spirit, but from the ground of implications and assumptions upon which appearance presents itself.


## BEAUTY IN PERCEPTION: MAKING AND KNOWING

The paradigm of beauty as appearance calls for a sense of beauty as vision itself. Plato refers to sight as "the keenest mode of perception vouchsafed us through the body" (*Phae.* 250 d). The aesthetic vision does not imply pure mirroring, because it entails the *joining* of two worlds, that of the seer and that of the seen, making or producing a third world in image. Gadamer understood beauty to be that which exists *between* idea and appearance.[33] This in-between state of *methexis* or coparticipation is the image. The perception of image, then, is the presencing of idea in appearance.

The sense of "making" in perception bespeaks the poetic basis of mind underlying the paradigm of beauty as appearance. The notion of the poetic basis of mind regards all mental activity as perception, i.e., what we are thinking and feeling is a matter of how we are seeing. It also considers all perception as inherently creative, i.e., each perception is the creation of a world. James Hillman writes:

Fantasy-images are both the raw materials and finished products of psyche, and they are the privileged mode of access to knowledge of soul. Nothing is more primary. Every notion in our minds, each perception of the world and sensation in ourselves must go through a psychic organization in order to happen at all. Every single feeling or observation occurs as a psychic event by first forming a fantasy-image.[34]

The Platonic tradition contributes to this paradigm through its sense of seeing as an action of procreation. In the *Symposium,* Socrates' notion that love is the desire for beauty is refined by Diotima. Diotima declares that love is not the longing for beauty but for the procreation that the beautiful effects. "To love is to bring forth upon the beautiful, both in body and in soul" (*Sym.* 206 b). (It is male and female, Diotima and Socrates together, who give expression to Plato's notion of love, as if in the act of conceiving.) Procreation involves the birth of a spark of the divine in matter. When this spark nears beauty, "it grows genial and blithe," and birth follows easily. When it nears the ugly, "it is overcome with heaviness and gloom, and turning away it shrinks into itself (*Sym.* 206 d). What soul longs for, then, is procreation, and this is what the beautiful effects. Beauty becomes like a midwife presiding over the soul's emergence in expression or image. My reading of Plato is that the vision of beauty joins the soul with appearance in a conjunction of love, and in the perceiving, image is both created and revealed. In sum, love of beauty effects a making, a creation of image. The hierarchical nature of the Neoplatonic universe insures that the making is effected, each level reproducing its own kind to form a subsequent level. "Everywhere a wisdom presides at a making" (*En.* V.8.5).

For Plotinus, literal action is a mode used by those who are weak in the ability to "see" in the contemplative mode. "They are left with a void because they cannot adequately seize the vision" (*En.* III.8.4). Plotinus does not consider action and vision as opposed. "Everywhere, doing and making will be found to be either an attenuation or a complement of vision" (*En.* III.8.4). Each envisioning is also making.

Plotinus follows Plato in his images of carpenters and weavers as the makers of the world. When one is reflecting, envisioning, or con-templating, one is making one's world through image making. One is crafting and shaping as does the creator of a statue that is to be made beautiful. One "cuts away here, he smooths there, he makes this line lighter, this one purer, until a lovely face has grown upon his work" (*En.* I.6.9). Seeing is a form of sculpting, the imagining eye shaping a world, creation coming into being with vision. "All the forms of

Authentic Existence spring from vision and are a vision. . . . Whatever exists is a bye-work of visioning" (*En.* III.8.7–8). All action in the
world springs from a ground of vision; how we see determines what
we do.

For Plotinus, the soul that has gone through the mysteries of beauty
to achieve a vision of the beauty beyond beauty, becomes vision itself.

> He that has known must love and reverence It as the very beauty; he will
> be flooded with awe and gladness, stricken by a salutary terror. . . . when
> you find yourself wholly true to your *essential nature,* wholly that only
> veritable Light which is not measured by space, not narrowed to any
> circumscribed form nor again diffused as a thing void of term, but ever
> unmeasurable as something greater than and more than all quantity—
> when you perceive that you have grown to this, you are now *become very
> vision:* now call up all your confidence, strike forward yet a step—you need
> a guide no longer—strain and *see.* (*En.* I.6.7–9) (Italics mine)[35]

The soul "become vision" is the process of psychological seeing—
seeing through the dualism of both literalism and representationalism
to the core of each appearance and happening. It is to see world
existing in vision, or as Blake writes, to see a "World in a Grain of
Sand."[36]

The images of impassioned movement and creativity in Plato and
Plotinus in relation to the aesthetic vision provide for a sense of action
in seeing. The action is contemplative rather than overt and has a
loving quality rather than one of control. The aesthetic vision, then,
would not only honor but care for appearance, considering perception
and the images of its own creation as one and the same.


## BEAUTY AND KNOWLEDGE

In Heidegger's reading of the *Phaedrus,* man is the "essence" to
which sentient beings reveal themselves in being.[37] This is possible
because the human soul alone has seen true 'being.' This view of being,
however, lies concealed in physical life. It is the erotic power of the
beautiful, shining through fleeting appearance that evokes thinking
about being. It is beauty in the immediacy of appearance that allows
for a vision of being's truth. In this sense, the aesthetic vision is a
means of knowing.

Following Heidegger, I see the Neoplatonic tradition as presenting
the apprehension of the beautiful as a way of thinking, *aisthesis* and
cognition coming together. Passing through the mysteries of beauty
allows for thought that sees. In this way, knowing and sensing would

not be different. Knowledge becomes accessible to what Hillman calls "thought of the heart,"[38] that thought which "joins with" in *eros* and "sees through," widening and deepening vision to reveal true being. What was once simply the seduction of the physical world becomes something more, a world of meaning or knowledge in appearance. Truth would then be seen in the sensual, what is there, the barefaced facts, or the facts of the bare face of the world.

Knowledge as aesthetic perception would not be something remote, to be derived through method, so much as a matter of memory, a recollection of form already there. The sense of knowledge as memory is most readily accessible in Plato's account in the *Phaedrus* of the soul's remembrance of its pre-earthly state.

> For only the soul that has beheld truth may enter into this our human form—seeing that man must needs understand the language of forms (*eidos*), passing from a plurality of perceptions to unity gathered together by reasoning—and such understanding is a recollection of those things which our souls beheld aforetime as they journeyed with their god, looking down upon the things which we now suppose to be, and gazing up to that which truly is. (*Phae.* 249 b–c)

In this statement that Plato gives Socrates, human understanding is characterized as a "gathering" of "perceptions" (*aisthesis*), that which is made present to the senses. According to John Sallis's commentary, it is understanding according to *eidos,* the *eidos* being the unity into which the perceptions are gathered.[39] *Eidos* is presumed to be prior in some way to the many perceptions. The priority of the *eidos* comes from the prior experience of the soul in its divine state in witnessing the ideal forms.

> Beauty it was ours to see in all its brightness in those days when amidst that happy company, we beheld with our eye that blessed vision; . . . pure was the light that shone around us. (*Phae.* 250 b)

In other words, the beauty of the world is close enough to heavenly beauty to remind the soul of the truth and wisdom of heavenly beauty. "As soon as he (the lover) beholds the beauty of the world, [he] is reminded of true beauty" (*Phae.* 249 e).

In sum, earthly perceptions, reminding the soul of the divine forms through their beauty, are gathered together in the service of the *eidos* that is akin to the divine form. These perceptions are shaped into image through the organizing influence of the *eidos.* The image brings about the memory of the truth of these perceptions. Acquisition of knowledge, then, is a matter of memory through beauty.

In Plotinus's model, the soul "free of body" attains the "Realm of Intellectual-Principles." "Wisdom is but the Act of the Intellectual-Principle withdrawn from the lower places and leading the Soul to the Above" (*En*. I.6.6). Here, the soul becomes "all Idea and Reason" (*En*. I.3.6). "Soul heightened to the Intellectual-Principle is beautiful to all its power. For Intellection and all that proceeds from Intellection are the Soul's beauty, a graciousness native to it and not foreign, for only with these is it truly Soul" (*En*. I.6.6). Thus, Plotinus imagines knowing as a realm, a way of being or a way of seeing in which truth is revealed. For Heidegger, this is *Dasein* as the "place" (*Da*) of the openness of being (*Sein*). This realm derives directly from the One and "is pre-eminently the manifestation of Beauty" (*En*. I.6.6). Beauty and the truth of the intellectual-principles are identical.

In other words, when we are really seeing the truth of something, it is due to the power of beauty that reveals such a truth. Truth brings the soul to its fullest beauty, and beauty brings the soul to its most complete truth. Beauty is an essential aspect of psychological knowing.


## THE AESTHETICS OF LIGHT

The notion of light is essential for a paradigm of beauty as appearance because it is light that allows for the display of appearance— no light, no perception, no knowledge, no being. It is the dispersal of light that allows for particularities to shine forth, each aspect perceivable in its own light revealing its own truth.

The idea of light as the wisdom of the divine has an ancient history. The semitic Baal, the Egyptian Ra, the Persian Mazda, Aphrodite, the Platonic Sun, and the *lumen naturae,* or fiery sparks of the world soul in alchemy, all give evidence to the sense of light's divinity. The most poetic and profound illustration of the aesthetics of light in Western literature is Dante's *Paradiso* in which the play of light is the major image of God.[40]

In the Platonic tradition, if love is the dynamic that brings *logos* out of estrangement and alienation, it is the principle of light that allows for its revealing through image. In the *Phaedrus* (250 c), Plato uses the word *ekphanestaton* (radiance) to mean "manifest to sense." What properly shows itself and is most radiant of all is the beautiful. It is light's "stream of beauty" (*Phae*. 251 b) that can animate the earthly soul. (The word *phaedrus* means "bright" or "beaming.")

Gadamer writes in his account of beauty in the *Phaedrus,* "The beautiful is truly 'most radiant' out of itself."[41] He explains that the "radiance" of beauty is the shining of light on something so that it is

able to appear. This light is not the light of the sun but the light of the mind, *nous*. Etymologically, beauty is related to the German *einleuch-tend*, "clear shining."

> The *eikos*, the verisimile, the 'probable' *wahrscheinliche*, literally 'true shining,' the 'clear,' belong in a series that defends its own rightness against the truth and certainty of what is proved and known.[42]

Gadamer's insight into Plato's notion of beauty shows that in radi-ance is revealing (*aletheia*). It is in the nature of form itself to reveal the truth of its own way. And in this revealing,

> the beautiful, the way in which goodness appears, reveals itself in its being, presents itself. What presents itself in this way is not different from itself in presenting itself.[43]

It is the radiance of each form that constitutes the actual being of beauty. It is light that allows the truth of each thing and event to reveal itself by shining through to perception.

> Indeed, just as the beautiful is a kind of experience that stands out like an enchantment and an adventure within the whole of our experience and presents a special task of hermeneutical integration, what is clear is always something surprising as well, like the turning on of a new light extending the range of what is to be taken into account.[44]

For Plotinus, the importance of the nature of beauty as light is in the movement away from beauty as form ("the primary nature of Beauty is formless," *En.* VI.7.33). Beauty, as the play of light throughout the universe, provides unity and the flexibility or flux of being. Beauty is not the static structure of symmetry (*En.* I.6.1), nor is it merely an attribute. Rather, it is an omnipresent principle of radiance "that is perceived at the first glance, something which the Soul names as from his ancient knowledge and, recognizing it, welcomes it, and enters into unison with it" (*En.* I.6.2).

The Christian Neoplatonic tradition saw light as a fundamental aspect of the nature of God.[45] One of the greatest of the Christian devotees of beauty as light was Dionysius the Areopagite (fifth and sixth centuries A.D.). Dionysius considered beauty as a name for God. He imagined light as the emanation of "Divine Goodness," radiating throughout the world.

> From the Good comes the light which is an image of Goodness; wherefore

the Good is described by the name of "light" being the archetype thereof which is revealed in that image.[46]

Dionysius saw in light not only the pervasive quality of the divine, each particular form honored through its radiance, but the simplicity of that which is fundamental as well.

This great, all-bright and ever-shining sun which is the visible image of the Divine Goodness faintly re-echoing the activity of the good, illumines all things that can receive its light while retaining the utter simplicity of light and expands above and below through the visible world the beam of its own radiance.[47]

In Ficino's cosmology, the force and heat of light is the fundament and cohesion of the universe.

Beauty is a certain act or ray from it [The Good] penetrating through all things. . . . It adorns the Mind with the order of Ideas. It fills the Soul with the series of the Reasons. It supports Nature with Seeds. It ornaments Matter with the Forms. But just as a single ray of the sun lights up four bodies, fire, air, water, and earth, so a single ray of God illumines the Mind, the Soul, Nature, and Matter. And just as anyone who sees the light in those four elements is looking at a ray of the sun itself and, through that ray is turned to looking at the supreme light of the sun, so anyone who looks at and loves the beauty in those four, Mind, Soul, Nature, and Body, is looking at and loving the splendor of God in them, and, through this splendor, God himself.[48]

For Ficino, the light of the heavens provides for human knowledge, *ratio lucis,* the reason of light. This is an image of the fruitfulness of life, the perspicacity of our senses, the penetration of our intelligence, and the bountifulness of grace. As Tom Moore notes, in his notion of *ratio luci* Ficino is placing soul as central in his cosmology.[49] Through light, the fantasies of soul permeate reason, so that the rational is contained in the psychological.

Psychologically, the aesthetics of light is important because it allows for a valuing of the particularity of each phenomenon.[50] Etymologically, the word *phenomenon,* an event experienced through the senses, has its roots in the word *phos* or light. A phenomenon, then, is that which shows itself through light. In every thing and every event there is a spark of divinity, a unique life that is connected to universal life. Beauty as radiance makes each earthly soul accessible to animation by the divine spark of life. Dionysius wrote:

But the Super-Essential Beautiful is called "Beauty" because of that quality

which it imparts to all things severally *according to their nature* and because It is the cause of the harmony and splendour in all things, flashing forth upon them all, like light, the beautifying communications of Its originating ray; and because It *summons all things,* to fare onto Itself (from whence It hath the name of "Fairness,") and because It *draws all things together* in a state of mutual interpenetration. (Italics mine.)[51]

For Plotinus, each soul possesses a faculty that is oriented toward beauty, a particular fragment of divine beauty that lies within. "Never can the Soul have vision of the First Beauty unless itself be beautiful" (*En.* I.6.9). Each individual soul is predisposed to receive the principle of beauty, welcoming and entering into communion with it. Plotinus anticipates psychotherapy, in that honoring particularity through light leads to the love of self by each particular being. "Anyone, unable to see himself, has but to bring the divine within before his consciousness and at once sees an image of himself, himself lifted to a better beauty" (*En.* V.8.2). Realizing one's own beauty is equivalent to "find[ing] yourself wholly true to your essential nature" (*En.* I.6.9).

Ficino saw the revelation of God in each particularity. "Thus," he says, "we are attracted to a certain man as a part of the world order especially when the spark of divine beauty shines brightly in him."[52] Each particular form has its own perfection.

This ray [the single ray of the one God] passes through angels, souls, the heavens and others' bodies. . . . Its splendor shines in every *individual thing according to its nature* and is called grace and beauty. (Italics mine.)[53]

As an idea in itself, Beauty ornaments every piece of matter with its own nature. Whereas Ficino would say that nothing is contemptible in the eye of God, the aesthetic psychologist would say that every appearance is a reflection of an archetype.

The aesthetics of light is also important for psychology because it gives an image for the relativizing of consciousness. For Ficino, although every form has its beauty, some forms are more available to beauty than others. Beauty is a quality of grace received by an object according to, among other factors, its "aspect" or shape and color.[54] In Jung's notion of "shadow," there is an image of the personal unconsciousness that provides shadings of value.[55] Through the play of light, then, perception is not all-or-nothing, black and white. Rather, it carries tones and shadings of emphasis and values that we give to everyday things and events.

In summary, the aesthetics of light paradoxically grounds the unique particularity of each part of the universe, each aspect perceivable in its own light, while giving rise to the "uni-tary" sense of the universe. It

allows for the radiance of knowledge as well as the darkness of ignorance. The play of light permits flexibility and relativizing of consciousness, as well as the perception of truths.

## BEAUTY AND THE ONE: UNITY, GOODNESS, AND BEING

I have emphasized the importance of particularity in beauty, but so also does experience include a sense of the unitary, eternal nature of the cosmos. I have emphasized the fluidity and flux of experience; but so also is there a fixed quality in being. I have emphasized the imme-diacy of experience; but so also does experience include a sense of the unseen or unknown goal. The unity, fixity, and goal-directed nature of beauty as appearance leads to the notion of beauty as the essence of being. As Hannah Arendt states in the quote that begins this book, being and appearing coincide. The appearing image becomes the pri-mary unit of psychological data or the ground of experience. We exist because we appear, because we are seen; and the power that allows for this appearance is beauty.

In the Neoplatonic tradition, the multiplicities of the universe are held together by the unity of the divine source. The unitary nature of the cosmos is prefigured by Heraclitus when he says, "The Logos is common to all."[56] It is beauty that allows for the unity of the universe and, as such, structurally lies in the proximity of goodness (fixity) and being itself.

For Plato, "the very soul of beauty" (Sym. 210 e) is the omnipresent element in all beings, the unity that expresses itself in diversity, the oneness that exists in and of itself.

> It is an everlasting loveliness which neither comes nor goes, which neither flowers nor fades, for such beauty is the same on every hand, the same then as now, here as there, this way as that way, the same to every worshipper as it is to every other.
>
> Nor will his vision of the beautiful take the form of a face, or of hands, or of anything that is of the flesh. It will be neither words, nor knowledge, nor something that exists in something else, such as a living creature, or the earth, or the heavens, or anything that is—but subsisting of itself and by itself in an eternal oneness, while every lovely thing partakes of it in such sort that, however much the parts may wax and wane, it will be neither more nor less, but still the same inviolable whole. (Sym. 211 a–b)

Plotinus situates beauty in the proximity of the ultimate One, the source of all life. The One is the "Authentic Beauty," "Beyond

Beauty," or "the First" (*En.* VI.7.33). It is the standard for the beauty of all existence. "This, then is Beauty primally; it is entire and omni-present as an entirety; and therefore in none of its parts or members lacking in beauty" (*En.* V.8.8).

> Its beauty, too will be unique, a beauty above beauty: it cannot be beauty since it is not a thing among things. It is loveable and the author of beauty; as the power to all beautiful shape, it will be the ultimate of beauty, that which brings all loveliness to be; it begets beauty and makes it yet more beautiful by the excess of beauty streaming from itself, the source and height of beauty. As the source of beauty it makes beautiful whatsoever springs from it. (*En.* VI.7.32)

Likewise for Dionysius, "the Beautiful" is unchangeable, eternal, and undying, the same for all parts, omnipresent over time and place, beautiful in relation to all, beheld by all as beautiful, unique in its beauty, and the originating source of all beauty.

> And it is called "Beautiful" because It is All-Beautiful and more than Beautiful and is eternally unvaryingly, unchangeably Beautiful; incapable of birth or death or growth or decay; and not beautiful in one part and foul in another; not yet at one time and not at another; nor yet beautiful in relation to one thing but not to another; nor yet beautiful in one place and not in another (as if It were beautiful for some but were not beautiful for others); nay, on the contrary, It is, in Itself and by Itself, uniquely and eternally beautiful, and from beforehand It contains in a transcendent manner the originating beauty of everything that is beautiful.[57]

The emphasis on unity in this aspect of the Neoplatonic tradition indicates an absolute, ultimate quality in beauty. Beauty appears as that which is the same in every instance of itself in which it is presented. It is always everywhere. It subsists in and of itself, and "every lovely thing partakes of it," even those that "wax and wane." Beauty is the ultimate source, above all distinctions, bestowing the unique perfection or soul inherent in the appearance of each event or thing. Psychologically speaking, beauty, as absolute, without time and space, brings together all contradictions. Through a sense of beauty we find light in the dark, black in the white, circle in the square. In short, beauty takes us out of oppositional seeing so that the logically paradox-ical becomes possible. Through beauty one comes to perceive and think in a unified way.

Beauty unifies the cosmos in that the beautiful is so, in some sense, to one and all. Without beauty, all beings would be in their own world. Through beauty, we recognize in the expressions of others that which is in our own experience. Beauty, as absolute, gives us our sense

of commonality, of community, making the world common ground for all.

The ultimate nature of beauty allows for the sense of *telos* or goal in experience. The qualities of absolute being in the Platonic universe—uniformity, unconditionality, boundlessness, permanence—are the qualities that make up the good, or "being as it ought to be" in Gadamer's words.[58] The tendency toward the congruence of beauty and the good is prefigured in Heraclitus. "To God all things are beautiful, good and right; men on the other hand, deem some things right and others wrong."[59] *Ekphanestaton,* which is "the radiance," and *phanotaton,* which is the good, both are derived from *phaiesthai,* "to appear" and "to shine forth." Following Gadamer's reading of Plato, the beautiful is related to the good, but distinguishable in that, unlike the good, the beautiful "can be laid hold of."[60] Plato asserts through Socrates in the *Philebus* (64e), "the good has taken refuge in the beautiful." In housing the good, the beautiful, through its own light and radiance, disposes the soul toward it. Through the soul's search for the good, the beautiful reveals itself. In the *Symposium,* good is the goal to which beauty leads.

> And remember, she [Diotima] said, that it is only when he discerns beauty itself through what makes it visible that a man will be quickened with the true, and not the seeming virtue—for it is virtue's self that quickens him, not virtue's semblance. And when he has brought forth and reared this perfect virtue, he shall be called the friend of god, and if ever it is given to man to put on immortality, it shall be given to him. (*Sym.* 212 a)

Ficino also identifies beauty as being near the good. He locates beauty as the central term in the three-fold nature of God: good, beautiful, the Just (truth). Beauty stands between goodness and justice, so that goodness and truth are witnessed in their splendor as beauty. Goodness shines forth as beauty, and beauty is the "splendor of the Good sparkling in the series of the ideas."[61] In summary, response to that which appears beautiful is response to beauty as an idea in itself, to the truth of all ideas and to goodness as the idea above all others.

Beauty, then, is the ground of being.[62] Heidegger reads the *Phaedrus* to say that the truth essentially brings about the unveiling of ultimate being. For Plotinus, being needs an image of beauty in order to present itself forth.

> Beauty without Being could not be, not Being voided of beauty: abandoned of Beauty, Being loses something of its essence. Being is desirable because it is identical with Beauty; and Beauty is loved because it is Being. . . . The

very figment of Being needs some imposed image of Beauty to make it possible. (*En.* V.8.9).

Dionysius also considered the ground of being to be the Beautiful. "From this Beautiful all things possess their existence, each kind being beautiful in its own manner."[63] All things and events possess their own unique being through Beauty. Beauty is the course of being, "all that is comes from the Beautiful and the Good,"[64] and the end, the "Goal of all things."[65] In sum, as Heidegger wrote, "The essence of the beautiful is what makes possible the recovery and preservation of the view of Being which devolves from the most immediate fleeting appearances."[66] In this view, being and appearance are one; we are because we appear.

## THE LIMITS OF THE PARADIGM OF BEAUTY AS APPEARANCE

Beauty as light is itself an image. Image both reveals and conceals, contains both truth and deceit.[67] Wherever light appears, behind it and to the side lies the dark in shades of gray and black. Jung used an aesthetic term for this inevitable blindness—the shadow. Hillman elaborates:

> For every bit of light that we grasp out of archetypal ambivalence, illumining with the candle of our ego a bright circle of awareness, we also darken the remainder of the room. At the same moment that we light the candle we create 'outer darkness', as if the light were a theft from the penumbra of dawn and twilight of paradoxical archetypal light.[68]

Rilke wrote in a letter:

> Like the moon, so life surely has a side that is constantly turned away from us, and that is not its opposite but its completion to perfection, to plentitude, to the real, whole and full sphere and globe of being.[69]

Around all of our little projects and projections lies the open and boundless dark.

If it is image or light or appearance or beauty that constitutes the primary realm of human experience or that establishes the ground of truth's possibility or that makes being manifest, then we live *in* image, appearance, light, or beauty and therefore can't know it. Our blindness is that we think *we* are seeing, when it is image, appearance, light, or beauty that is seeing *through* us. Ultimately, what unites us is not our

seeing, but that which we can't see, because it makes consciousness possible in the first place. Like the dying Goethe, we want "more light," but paradoxically, it is in the darkness that we find our home. Hillman quotes Lao Tzu: "Soften the light, become one with the dusty world."[70]

PART TWO
# BEAUTY AS INTERIOR EXPERIENCE

# APHRODITE REFUSED

When Augustine inquired about the nature of God, he asked the various things of the world, and they replied, "I am not he." Augustine wrote in his *Confessions,* "My questioning was in my contemplation of them and their answer was in their beauty."[1] The things of the world, giving answer through their beauty, provide an Aphrodisian image, the divine shining through the particularities of the world. Augustine sang a song of praise to beauty, "Late it was that I loved you, beauty so ancient and so new, late I loved you!"[2]

Yet beauty for Augustine was not the beauty of Aphrodite, appearance as goddess. Augustine's focus was toward inner life.

> And look, you were within me and I was outside and there I sought for you and in my ugliness I plunged into the beauties that you have made. You were with me and I was not with you. . . . You called, you cried out, you scattered my deafness: you flashed, you shone, you scattered my blindness: You breathed perfume, and I drew in my breath and I pant for you.[3]

Light and perfume are attributes of Aphrodite, and the entire lyric is one of Aphrodisian desire. However, the ultimate object of Augustine's love was not of the earth but the heavens. The call from the heavens is a spiritual calling, and beauty within was Augustine's link to God.

This chapter is meant to serve as an introduction to the paradigm of beauty as internal process, in that it is about the turning of consciousness inward, away from appearance, toward spiritual and conceptual experience. My purpose in the chapter will not be to devalue spirit or concept, but to indicate how spirit and reason in the service of spirit can lead to a devaluing of appearance. Psyche needs spirit for its sense of order, precision, discrimination, and focus. Ficino thought of spirit as a mediator between soul and world, a form of nourishment for soul. From a perspective of psyche as the middle ground of spirit and matter, however, it is important to maintain the sense of spirit as dwelling within appearance, as well as within faith and concept.

In this chapter, I shall attempt to introduce the paradigm of beauty

as an internal process by illustrating the turn away from appearance in early Christian and in Protestant consciousness. In subsequent chap-ters, I will show how, separated from appearance itself, beauty be-comes a matter of concept (proportion), which becomes literalized into an understanding of the world through method (linear perspective) and finally is subjectivized so that it becomes separate from knowledge. I will also try to show how the psychological effect of this progression in Western consciousness—beauty as spiritual experience, concept, method, subjective experience—is an increased emphasis on control, certainty, and identification with divine perspective in the subject. The ultimate result is the diminishment in value of beauty as an objective reality.

Elaine Pagels, E. R. Dodds, and Hannah Arendt all remark upon the shift in consciousness away from the body and the world toward interiority in the early Christian age.[4] Pagels suggests that this turn on the part of early Christians is in the service of *autexousia,* a notion of personal freedom from necessity. She writes that until Augustine, Christians regarded personal freedom as the primary message of Gene-sis. *Autexousia* included free will, freedom from government and fate, and freedom from sexual obligation. This freedom was brought about through self-mastery of emotions and desires. Pagels quotes Gregory of Nyssa:

> The soul immediately shows its royal and exalted character . . . in that it owns no master and is self governed, ruled autocratically by its own will.[5]

Augustine interpreted Genesis differently, reading in it the story of human bondage to sexuality. Ever since the Fall, freedom of will had been lost. Spontaneous sexual desire was both proof and penalty of original sin. Government, especially in the form of the Church, was necessary as a defense against the power of bodily desire.

In both doctrines, the freedom of will and the necessity of the Church as protector against spontaneous sexuality, the body was considered as alien, and consciousness was oriented away from the body and hence from the world. In regard to the turn from the world by pagans and Christians alike, Dodds recalls the influence of the pagan notion of the earth as dark, cold, and impure in comparison to the light, warmth, and purity of the heavens. In this tradition, matter is a source of evil, embodiment a form of exile, and human existence an alien, unnatural condition. The result is a turn by consciousness away from body and world in the service of an introverted quest for spiritual being.

The turn from matter was paralleled by a shift in consciousness

away from appearance. Arendt cites the change in attitude toward appearance that came about with the apostle Paul and with the Stoic Epictetus.

> Hence, when we come to Paul, the accent shifts entirely from doing to believing, from the outward man living in a world of appearances (himself an appearance among appearances and therefore subject to semblance and illusion) to an inwardness which by definition never unequivocally man-ifests itself and can be scrutinized only by a God who also never appears unequivocally.[6]

Arendt considers the turn inward to be in the service of the concept of will. She writes, "In each [Paul and Epictetus], the actual content of inwardness is described exclusively in terms of the promptings of the Will, which Paul believed to be impotent and Epictetus declared to be almighty."[7]

Looking closely at Arendt's analysis, there are three themes at work in the movement toward interiority in the service of the will—identifi-cation with the divine, control, and certainty. Arendt suggests that for both the early Christians and the Stoics the turn away from the physical world was in response to a need for identification with immortality. Denial of the body and of the transience of earthly life is the denial of limits that death imposes on mortal being. The movement of consciousness inward also gives humanity a sense of control in that if we are independent of the influence of the harsh, physical world, we are free from fear of pain or death. When bodily existence is acknowl-edged, man is rendered dependent on the environment. With the movement toward interiority, outside influences become mere mental impressions that can be controlled by the mind. Arendt paraphrases Epictetus:

> The power of the will rests on its sovereign decision to concern itself only with things within man's power, and these reside exclusively in human inwardness. . . . Everything that seems to be real, the world of appearance, actually needs my consent in order to be real *for me.* And this consent cannot be forced on me: if I withold it, then the reality of the world disappears as though it were a mere apparition.[8]

Finally, whereas appearance always raises the specter of deception, the movement inward lends itself to a sense of certainty. Independent of the flux of outer life, the mind can not be deceived. Free of the deceptive influence of the physical world, life becomes "the soundless, swift dialogue of the mind's exchange with itself, an exchange whose

very 'sweetness' consists in a spirituality in which no material factor intervenes."[9]

The rejection of appearance and its replacement with a conceptual and spiritual orientation is evident in the attack by some early Christian fathers upon Aphrodite as goddess of sexual love. For those Christians who zealously attempted to teach the ways of the spirit, Aphrodite as voluptuous goddess of form was a demon, "the overseer of intercourse," and the most shameful of the Olympian gods.[10] In the Christian imagination, love implied not sexual love in the name of fertility, but spiritual love of God. The polytheistic sense of love and beauty as a goddess became the logocentric sense of God as love; love of God came to be celebrated over human love between the sexes. Gregory the Great is said to have declared, "The sirens have the faces of women because nothing estranges men from God as much as the love of women."[11] Dodds notes in the Sentences of Sextus, an early Christian writing, the idea that marriage should be a "competition in continence" and that self-castration was a preferable alternative. In addition he reminds us of Paul's assertion that only virgins would be resurrected.[12]

Constantine, who in 313 B.C. became the first Christian emperor of Rome, raided the shrines of Aphrodite wherein sacred prostitution was performed. Eusebios, a follower of Constantine, described one temple as

> a hidden and fatal snare of souls dedicated to the foul demon known by the name of Aphrodite. . . . Here men undeserving of the name forgot the dignity of their sex and propitiated the demon by their effeminate conduct: here too, unlawful commerce with women and adulterous intercourse with other horrific and infamous practices were perpetrated.[13]

Arnobius of Sicca wrote in "The Case Against the Pagans" of the "evil deeds" of the goddess.

> For if, as you assert and believe, she enkindles the flames of love in human minds, one must then understand that to the wounds of Venus must be attributed whatever disgrace or misdeed arises from such madness. Is it, therefore, under compulsion from the goddess that even the noble frequently surrender their honor to harlots of the worst repute; that the firm ties of marriage gradually loosen; that relationship by blood is inflamed [toward] incestuous passions; that mothers nurture a mad love for their children; that fathers turn to themselves the longings of their daughters; that flouting the dignity that goes with their age, old men are filled with youthful passions for filthy gratifications; that wise and brave men, living in dissipation of the sinews of their manhood, exchange the demands of

constancy for effeminacy: that people hang themselves; and, commonly enough, cast themselves—leaping deliberately from the heights of jagged cliffs.[14]

Arnobius goes on to decry the "filthy" morality of such a god and calls for the virtue of a god removed from emotion.

Clement of Alexandria wrote to the Greeks that worship of their gods took them down the "slippery and harmful paths which lead away from the truth, *dragging man down from heaven* and overturning him into the pit." (Italics mine.)[15] He asserted that the Greek gods were false in that they were mere mortals who had been raised to the status of deities. Evidence of this lay in the account of Aphrodite's wound in *The Iliad,* as well as the acts of laughter and sex in which the gods indulged. (Both of these latter activities are in the domain of Aphrodite.)

> How in the world is it that you have given credence to worthless legends, imagining brute beasts to be enchanted by music, while the bright face of truth seems alone to strike you as deceptive, and is regarded with unbelieving eyes?[16]

For Clement, the truth could only lay in God's word, *logos* as spiritual seed.

Aphrodite was a special target for Clement's invectives against the Greek gods.

> There is, then, the "foam-born" "Cyprisus-born" goddess, the darling of Cinyras. I mean Aphrodite, who received the name Philomedes because she was born from the *medea,* those lustful members that were cut off from Uranus and after the separation did violence to the wave. See how lewd are the members from which so worthy an offspring is born! And in the rites which celebrate this pleasure of the sea, as a symbol of her birth, the gift of a cake of salt and a *phallos* is made to those who are initiated in the art of fornication; and the initiated bring their tribute of a coin to the goddess, as lovers do to a mistress.[17]

Clement showed special disdain for the "lustful orgies" that took place in Aphrodite's temples as fertility rites.

> I must leave you to judge whether it is a respectable proceeding to prostrate yourselves to whores.[18]

> We read of Aphrodite, how like a wanton hussy she brought the stool for Helen, and placed it in front of her paramour in order that Helen might entice him to her arms.[19]

In recounting Homer's story of the love affair of Aphrodite and Ares, Clement cries out, "Cease the song, Homer. There is no beauty in that; it teaches adultery."[20]

Clement condemned attributes of Aphrodite other than her sex-uality. Aphrodite, as the goddess "of laughing eyes" and "she of the smiles," became the indirect object of Clement's attack on levity. "Men who imitate laughable or ridiculous behavior are to be excluded from the city—as for laughter itself, it too should be kept under restraint."[21] Whereas, Aphrodite was goddess of the realm of perfumes, odors, and decorations, Clement warns, "The use of wreathes and of perfumes is not a necessity for us. Rather, it shipwrecks us upon pleasure and frivolity even as night draws near."[22] For Clement, the lord offers the only gift of smell that matters, the scent of his love. Unguents should only be used for utilitarian purposes. Clement is strict about embellish-ment of any kind—"gaudiness, the dying of wool, variegation of colors, elaborate jewelry, ornamentations, gold, wigs, eye-shadow, make up, hair dye and all artifices to make us appear what we are not."[23] Likewise, precious stones incur Clement's scorn: It is pure childishness to let ourselves become fascinated by gems, whether they are green or dark red, and by the stones disgorged by the sea, and by the metals dug up out of the earth.[24] Appearance is not to be trusted. "Surely we should uproot all love for ornamentation, for it contributes nothing to the growth of virtue, but instead pampers the body."[25]

Finally Clement condemns the many statues of Aphrodite and the art of sculpting itself. He deplores the legends of Pygmalion and the man who had intercourse with the Cnidian statue of Aphrodite. These stories gave Clement evidence of the demonic nature of both Aphro-dite and the art of sculpture, implanting "insane passion" in humanity, rendering us beneath even the monkey in the ability to discriminate.[26] For Clement, the only true image, the image of God, is borne within.

Thus, the early Christian fathers worked to displace a sensual orientation associated with the worship of Aphrodite with an ex-clusively spiritual orientation toward experience.

The ambivalence regarding image within the medieval Church can be seen in the history of the conflict surrounding iconoclasm. In this conflict the question of whether or not spirit could be venerated as infused in matter was addressed.[27] Christians in the Greek-speaking and eastern areas of the Byzantine Empire perpetuated their earlier tradition of the use of images through the veneration of icons. That part of the Christian world founded upon the Semitic tradition of faith in a God without images objected to this practice.

In 725 and 726 A.D., the Byzantine emperor Leo III initiated a policy

of iconoclasm in which veneration of images was banned and all images were ordered destroyed. Ironically, one of the images destroyed was that of Christ, set up by Constantine after he had destroyed sculptures of Aphrodite. Opposition by monks brought a wave of persecution that was to last for several years. John of Damascus wrote three apologies, which were together entitled *In Defense of the Sacred Images,* and Popes Gregory II and Gregory III protested, as did the Council of Rome.

Leo's son, Constantine V, furthered his father's measures by encouraging an iconoclastic doctrine that was enforced by the Council of Hiereia in 754. Iconoclastic theologians claimed that to represent the Savior in handmade material was to limit his divinity, which they held to be essentially indescribable. Proponents for icon veneration thought that icons were demonstrative of his incarnation. The persecutions continued until Irene, the widow of Leo IV and herself from a Greek region, assumed the regency in 780 and restored the cult of icon veneration. In 787 she convened the Second Council of Nicaea, which endorsed the veneration of images as "relative" worship— that is, icons were declared to be mediators to their divine prototypes. However, when Leo V was brought to the throne (through the efforts of the army that was opposed to icons), the Council of Hagia Sophia in 815 invalidated the decrees of 787 and recognized the doctrine of Hiereia (754). Finally, in 843, the assumption to the throne of another woman, Theodore, brought about the restoration of image veneration at another council in Constantinople. This council marked the conclusion of the iconoclastic crisis and there followed a long period in which icon production flourished in Byzantium.

The devaluation of beauty as appearance in the service of faith in spirit and reason is reflected in Protestantism as well as early Catholicism. Luther's sense of the primacy of individual faith lead him to assert that the soul is not affected by the outer world. He wrote, "It is evident that no external thing, whatsoever it be, has any influence whatever [on the soul]."[28] For Luther, all appearance of the outer world is deceptive; the soul can only take refuge in the word of God.

In like manner, the Aphrodisian themes of the proximity of the divine to humans and humanity's connection to the divine through love were rejected by Luther. Luther thought that God favored the one who would "agree" with God's judgment of humanity being distant from him and therefore sinful.[29] "It is not he who considers himself the most lowly of men but he who sees himself as even the most vile, who is most beautiful to God."[30] Salvation was brought about by "sheer" and "naked" faith, not love.[31] Thus, the idea that one could come to

know God by developing likeness (*simultudo*) to him through love (*caritas*) was completely rejected by Luther in favor of a spiritual attitude based upon pure faith.

In the Protestant mind, nature and spirit are irreconcilable, produc' ing a fundamental antagonism to sensuous culture. Richard Baxter (1615–91), "the chief of English Protestant schoolmen," wrote:

> Suppose with thyself thou hadst been that Apostle's fellow traveller into the celestial kingdom, and that thou hadst seen all the saints in their white robes, with palms in their hands; suppose thou hadst heard those songs of Moses and the Lamb; or didst even now hear them praising and glorifying the living God. If thou hadst seen these things indeed, in what a rapture wouldst though have been? I would not have thee, as the Baptists, draw them in pictures, nor use mysterious significant ceremonies to represent them. This, as it is a course forbidden by God, so it would but seduce and draw down thy heart; but get the liveliest picture of them in thy mind that possibly thou canst.[32]

The Protestant emphasis on interiority and the resulting devalua' tion of beauty as appearance presents itself in the poetry of John Milton. Milton's attitude toward appearance is reflected in his disparaging characterizations of Eve and Delilah, the personifications of feminine beauty. I would suggest that these two figures are degraded forms of Aphrodite in that they are embodiments of those themes once personified in the goddess—image, shape, body, and appearance. These notions are identified by Milton with the female gender and devalued as leading the male gender, representing reason, away from the primary task of spiritual faith.

Woman as sensuous appearance is infirm, beguiling, and deceiving of man, lax in his faith. The Chorus in *Samson Agonistes* presents the extreme of this view.

> What'ere it be, to wisest men and best
> Seeming at first all heavenly under virgin veil,
> Soft, modest, meek, demure,
> Once join'd, the contrary she proves, a thorn
> Intestine, far within defensive arms
> A cleaving mischief, in his way to virtue
> Adverse and turbulent, or by her charms
> Draw him awry enslav'd
> With dotage, and his sense deprav'd
> To folly and shameful deeds which ruin ends.

(SA 1034–43)

Delilah is depicted by the Chorus in the metaphorical image of a

ship, shifting her course with the courtship of any wind, drawing attention to herself through the superficial means of ornamentation and perfume rather than through the rectitude of the mind (SA 710–21). As "deceitful Woman" (SA 202), Delilah's infirmity is in her curiosity and inability to hold Samson's secret within, "both common female faults" (SA 776). She offers Samson love, but "Love seeks to have Love" (SA 837), instead of seeking the "highest wisdom" in God (SA 1747).

Samson's tragic fault lay in his abandonment of faith and reason for the pleasures of sensual life. His myth is that of the soul trapped in body, "Imprison'd now indeed, / In real darkness of the body" (SA 158–9), "exiled from light" (SA 97). In his blindness, Samson comes to discover and "see" the spirit within, and his regeneration rests in giving up earthly life for faith in God's justice.

In *Paradise Lost*, it is imagination, the faculty concerned with image, that leads humans astray, as opposed to reason, which leads us to God. Eve, the carrier of imagination and sensual life untempered by reason, is the cause of the Fall.

> For Understanding rul'd not, and the Will
> Heard not her lore, both in subjection now
> To sensual Appetite, who from beneath
> Usurping over sovran Reason claim'd
> Superior sway.
>
> (PL IX 1127–31)

For Milton, imagination is associated with Satan, through Eve, and reason is associated with God through Adam.[33] It is Satan who engenders "sensual Appetite," "Assaying by his Devilish art to reach / The Organs of her [Eve's] Fancy, and with them forge / Illusions as he list, Phantasms and Dreams" (Pl IV 801–3)." In a dream, it is the image of the forbidden tree of knowledge that lures Eve, "fair it seem'd, Much fairer to my Fancy than by day" (PL V 52–53), as a prefiguration of Satan's later leading her astray.

Eve's submission to the temptation of Fancy is prefigured by her confusion of her own image in the water with that of another person.

>                    I thither went
> With unexperienc't thought, and laid me down
> On the green bank, to look into the clear
> Smooth Lake, that to me seem'd another Sky.
> As I bent down to look, just opposite,
> A Shape within the wat'ry gleam appear'd
> Bending to look on me, I started back,

It started back, but pleas'd I soon return'd,
Pleas'd it return'd as soon with answering looks
Of sympathy and love; there I had fixt
Mine eyes till now, and pin'd with vain desire,
Had not a voice thus warn'd me.

(*PL* IV 456–66)

This allusion to the myth of Narcissus is a metaphorical depiction of the soul's mistaken fall into matter.[34] Again, appearance is associated with matter and therefore not to be trusted without the spiritualizing influence of reason. Faith in spirit, not appearance, engenders certainty.

The lesson of *Paradise Lost* is that imagination needs to be in the service of reason in order to serve the soul. Reason, the "chief" of the soul's faculties, shapes fancy and sensate data to form knowledge.

But know that in the Soul
Are many lesser Faculties that serve
Reason as chief; among these Fancy next
Her office holds; of all external things,
Which the five watchful Senses represent,
She forms Imaginations, Aery shapes,
Which Reason joining or disjoining, frames
All what we affirm or what deny, and call
Our knowledge or opinion.

(*PL* V 100–108)

Reason claims the male gender as its earthly sanctuary, making man "superior" to woman (*PL* IV 499).

though both
Not equal, as their sex not equal seem'd;
For contemplation hee and valor form'd,
For softness shee and sweet attractive Grace,
Hee for God only, shee for God in him.

(*PL* 295–301)

Adam's "fair large Front and Eye sublime declar'd / Absolute rule" (*PL* IV 300–301), while Eve's hair "Dishevell'd, but in wanton ringlets waved / . . . impli'd / Subjection" (*PL* IV 306–8). Eve herself confesses, "How beauty is excell'd by manly grace / And wisdom which alone is truly fair" (*PL* IV 490–91).

Eve, as woman, embodies the outer "charm of Beauty," but she lacks the inner excellence of reason.

Too much of Ornament, in outward show

Elaborate, of inward less exact.
For well I understand in the prime and
Of Nature her th' inferior, in the mind
And inward Faculties, which most excel.

                                        (PL VIII 538-42)

Reason, not Beauty, is what leads to God, "for what obeys / Reason is free, and Reason he made right" (PL IX 351–52).

Milton's most devastating image of beauty is the association of woman with the serpent. In *Paradise Lost,* Eve's luring of Adam to the tree of knowledge is prefigured in Sin's seduction of her father, Satan. Sin "seem'd Woman to the waist, and fair, / But ended foul in many a scaly fold / Voluminous and vast, and Serpent arm'd / With mortal sting" (PL II 650–53). In his despair Adam reminds Eve of her association with Satan as serpent and refers to her by that name:

Out of my sight, thou Serpent, that name best
Befits thee with him leagu'd, thyself as false
And hateful; nothing wants, but that thy shape,
Like his, and color Serpentine may show
Thy inward fraud.

                                        (PL 867–71)

Likewise the Chorus refers to Delilah "as manifest Serpent by her sting / Discovered in the end, till now conceal'd" (SA 997–98). Woman as serpent gives evidence to the sense of deceit, inconstancy, "inward fraud," and lethality that Milton associates with appearance. Beauty—she who was Golden Aphrodite, the appearance through which the world of the divine was made known to man, she through whom truth and goodness revealed themselves—is subordinated when the inner eye of reason dominates consciousness.

If Milton's Eve and Delilah are the images of Aphrodite devalued in relation to reason, three Renaissance paintings might be seen as para-digmatic images of the turn toward beauty as spirit. Kenneth Clark notes the change in Aphrodite revealed in the painting *The Temperance of Chastity* (1300–1310), by Giovani Pisano.

The means by which he has, so to say, Christianized the Venus is the turn and expression of the head. Instead of looking in the same direction as her body, and thus confirming her existance in the present, she turns and looks upward over her shoulders toward the promised world of the future. Her right arm, bent so that her hand comes higher on her breast and really covers it, lands the eye back to the head.[35]

The Mona Lisa has been regarded by J. H. Van Den Berg as the very

image of the smiling "inner self," the locus of animation entirely within the human figure, the face completely separate from the landscape behind.[36] The third image is Botticelli's work *Truth,* a female figure painted late in his career. Kenneth Clark comments that by this time Botticelli had lost his sense of the sensual body, and, instead of the classic curves of Venus, Truth is painted with her arms and the angle of her head in a "zig-zag diamond-shaped pattern."[37] In this triangular pattern one might see the image of dialectic, proportion, and linear perspective. These are the patterns of the paradigm of beauty as spirit that I shall explore in the next chapters.

In conclusion, the turn inward as reflected in one tradition of early Christianity, Stoicism, and Protestantism results in the loss of faith in image in favor of faith in spirit and reason. I am suggesting this to be a movement from one paradigm of beauty to another. In the next three chapters, I hope to show that this consciousness results not only in the decline of beauty as a principle, but in the identification of human perspective with the control and certainty of divine perspective.

# PROPORTION: BEAUTY AS MEASURE

The basis for the paradigm of beauty as an internal process is the concept of proportion. The fundamental principle of proportion is that concrete particularity is reducible to intelligible unity through order in the relationship of the parts. Proportion refers to the way the different parts of a whole come together, answering the question, "To what degree does the variety within a thing form a unity?" Beauty as proportion is based upon abstractions, that is, numerical properties, not what appears concretely to the senses. Proportion, then, is not strictly aesthetic, but metaphysic. Proportion has to do with quantity, as opposed to quality, concept, as opposed to image. Beauty as proportion lends itself to an inner-directed, transcendent consciousness, because the focus of attention is not what appears, manifest to sense, but a scheme of numerical order that is linked to the ideal and applied to appearance.

The sense of beauty as proportion existed throughout antiquity and became dominant in the Middle Ages. The ancient Egyptians developed a canon of proportion that Egyptian artisans used in sculpture for a wide range of purposes that extended from the establishment of dimensions to the definition of movement. A pre-Socratic Greek fragment states, "Order and proportion are beautiful and useful."[1] A fragment from Polyclitus says, "The beautiful comes about little by little, through many numbers."[2] Galen wrote:

> [Chrysippus] holds that beauty does not consist in the elements but in the harmonious proportion of the parts, the proportion of one finger to the other, of all the fingers to the rest of the hand, of the rest of the hand to the wrist, of these to the forearm, of the forearm to the whole arm, in fine, of all parts to all others, as it is written in the cannon of Polyclitus.[3]

Pythagorus (sixth century B.C.) was one of the earliest important theoreticians of proportion. He combined the two realms of mathematics and religion, a fact that reflects the spiritual foundation for the concept of proportion. Pythagorus was the leader of a religious order that believed that the human soul is immortal and is manifested in

many reincarnations. The goal in life is for the soul to transcend the prison of the body, thereby becoming pure spirit and rejoining the universal spirit to which it essentially belongs. Pythagorus believed that spiritual existence could be achieved through the inherent order in the universe and initiated the Greek term *kosmos,* which combines the notions of order, fitness, and beauty.[4]

The foundation of Pythagorus's belief in order was the emphasis he placed upon the idea of "limit" over the "unlimited." The imposition of limit *(peras)* upon the unlimited *(apeiron)* produced the limited *(peperasmenon).* By contemplating the principle of order through the imposition of limit upon the unlimited and by assimilating ourselves to that order, humanity becomes purified. In sum, for Pythagorus, the notions of contemplation, order, and purification were spiritual equiv-alents.

The ground for Pythagorus's sense of order through limit was his faith in numbers. Number imposes limit upon the unlimited. Pythagorus discovered that the intervals of the musical scale can be expressed arithmetically as the ratios between the numbers one, two, three, and four. The perfect number was the sum of these numbers, ten. (The Latin word for proportion, *consonatia,* means "sounding together.") Extrapolating from this discovery, Pythagoreans came to the conclusion that all things in the universe were ordered through numbers in the same way as the musical scale. The point was consid-ered as one, the line, two, the surface, three, and the solid, four. Each thing, like each sound, is what it is, not through how it appears, but through the distribution of its elements. In short, the Pythagoreans were convinced that "things were numbers."[5] What the Plotinian would see as differences in quality, Pythagoreans saw as differences in quantity.

In summary, for Pythagorus there is a clear association of number, order, limit, and spiritual purification. The contemplation of the order of numbers, in itself, makes one pure. Particularity is associated with the unlimited and the grossness of sensual appearance. Through con-templation as a spiritual discipline, the identity of things is trans-formed from one of sensuous characteristics to one of number.

For Plato, the good—that is, fixity, purity, and truth—is separate from the physical world. There are two avenues by which the good makes itself accessible, one following in the tradition of Homer, the other in the tradition of Pythagorus. The first, as seen in the *Phaedrus* and the *Symposium,* follows the tradition that is based upon the aesthetics of light. Beauty alone, of all the Forms, shines through to human perception. Beauty is an indefinable principle that supervenes upon the world. In this sense, beauty is not identical to the good;

rather, the good takes refuge in beauty (*Philebus* 64 e).[6] Beauty, as light manifest to sense and directly perceptible, leads to the Good.

Plato's second mode for access to the good lies in the tradition of Pythagorus in its utilization of measure.[7] The Pythagorean influence on Plato is most evident in regard to measure. In the *Republic* and the *Philebus*, Plato follows the Pythagoreans by distinguishing between the limited and the unlimited aspects of the universe. Socrates states, "We said, I fancy, that God had revealed two constituents of things, the unlimited and the limit" (*Phil.* 23 c). The mixture of the limited with the unlimited becomes "the source of . . . beautiful things" (*Phil.* 26 b). In this orientation, the beautiful is not light but moderation. The means for imposing moderation or limit on the unlimited is through number or measure.

> So now we find that the good has taken refuge in the character of the beautiful, for the qualities of measure and proportion invariable, I imagine, constitute beauty and excellence. (*Phil.* 64 e)

The "men of old," so Socrates relates (perhaps referring to Pythagoreans), say that only when one has grasped the "number and nature of the intervals formed by high and low pitch in sound," the "figures," and "measures," has one gained "real understanding" (*Phil.* 17 d–e). On the other hand, the unlimited form of understanding is associated with particulars and leaves one "an unlimited ignoramus" (*Phil.* 17 e). Particularity is associated with lack of limitation and, as such, has no value. Measure is the mixing of the limited and the unlimited and therefore leads to the good (*Phil.* 61 b, 65 a). The "first of possessions," Socrates concludes, is in the "region of measure" (*Phil.* 66 a).

Plato's model for the good as presented in the *Republic* is that it is a reality that gives truth to objects and the power of knowing to the knower.

> This reality, then, that gives their truth to the objects of knowledge and the power of knowing to the knower, you must say is the idea of the good, and you must conceive it as being the cause of knowledge, and of truth in so far as known. . . . An inconceivable beauty you speak of [i.e., the good], he said, if it is the source of knowledge and truth, and yet itself surpasses them in beauty. (*Rep.* VI 508 e–509 a)[8]

With this sense of beauty, Plato is emphasizing the proximity of beauty to the good as the source of truth and knowing and its distance from human perception. Therefore, the soul must be turned to this, the "brightest region of being" (*Rep.* VII 518c), through artificial means.

There are few who can apprehend the beauty of true being. Most people perceive as if seeing only shadows cast by the light of being shining from behind them. The eye of these persons must be turned around from the world of becoming to the world of being "until the soul is able to endure the contemplation of essence" (*Rep.* 518c). An art for the conversion of the soul is needed to help direct vision to the source. This art turns vision from the downward seduction of physical appearance to the upward vision that sees essence. The instruments for this purpose are number, geometry, astronomy, and dialectic. It is the ability of these sciences to deal in proportion that allows them to lead the eye away from sensual perception and to reveal pure knowledge (*Rep.* VII 530a). The sciences are tools that lead the mortal eye from concrete particularity to the unity of knowledge. In this paradigm, it is *methodology*, the procedures of the arts and sciences, rather than love, that leads the "best part of the soul up to the contemplation of what is best among realities" (*Rep.* 532c).

Augustine expanded the idea that beauty is based upon number into the metaphysics of proportion. For Augustine, participation in the unity of Divine will is possible through beauty, and beauty is possible through number. "Examine the beauty of bodily form," he wrote, "and you will find that everything is in its place by number."[9]

Number has several meanings for Augustine. First, it is mathematical proportion. "It is the proportion *numeri*, which is the source of pleasure."[10] Second, number is rhythmic organization.

> Those rhythms excel by virtue of the beauty of reason, which if we were cut off from them altogether when we incline towards the body, would cease to govern the Progressive Rhythm perceptible to sense, and to create perceptible beauties of temporal duration by bodily movement.[11]

Third, number is the fittingness of parts or *aequalitas*, equilibrium.

> Beautiful things please by proportion, *numero*, and here as we have shown, equality is not found only in sounds for the ear and in bodily movements, but also in visible forms, in which hitherto, equality has been identified with beauty. . . . Nothing can be proportionate or rhythmic, *numerosus*, without equality. . . . Where there is equality or similitude, there is rhythmicality, *numerositas*, for nothing is so equal or so similar to anything as one is to one.[12]

Finally, number in Augustine refers to the Divine. "When the soul has properly adjusted and disposed itself, and has rendered itself harmonious and beautiful, then will it venture to see God, the very source of all truth and the very Father of Truth."[13]

Augustine defines beautiful, not in terms of appearance, but in terms

of reason. Image, for Augustine, is a source of illusion. The man who "does not yield to images" is "most deserving of the attribute learned."[14] Instead, the beautiful is that in which "the harmony of parts is wont to be reason."[15] The beauty of reason "causes things to excell."[16] Augustine considers reason itself as animated, "nothing pleased it but beauty and in beauty, design, and in design, dimension, and in dimension, number."[17] Knowledge comes about through the "science of right reasoning and that of the power of numbers."[18] "It is not by making well measured things, but by grasping the nature of numbers that I am the more excellent."[19]

One of the most important aspects of Augustine's sense of beauty is that beauty is intricately related to equivalency or symmetry. In this notion, everything has an equal and opposite counterpart with which it is paired. Something is beautiful to the extent that it fits with another component. Nothing is considered in and of itself but always in relation to something else.

The importance of symmetry for Augustine can be seen in his hierarchy of geometric forms according to the equality of lines. With the principle of equivalency, a figure bounded by equal lines is more perfect and more beautiful than one without; therefore, an equilateral triangle is more perfect and more beautiful than a scalene triangle. Since the square has an equal number of sides, it is more perfect than the equilateral triangle. The circle is more perfect than the square because nothing interrupts its equality. The most excellent form of all is the point because it has no division and is inherently a unity.

Augustine's conception that the point is the most perfect of figures indicates his centristic orientation. In Augustine's conception of equiv' alency, not only must each form have a relationship to an equivalent form, but it must have a relationship to a center as well. "All that is single, singular, must have some central place, so that equality may be preserved in the intervals extending to the central individual part."[20] Augustine's emphasis on the center indicates the priority that he gives to unity over particularity. His view of Genesis, for example, was that only after the light, as unity, was formed could heaven and earth be shaped into the multiplicity of forms.[21]

If he (man) reduces to a simple, true and certain unity all the things that are scattered far and wide throughout so many branches of study, then he is most deserving of the attribute learned.[22]

In Augustine's sense, then, beauty is an attribute held only by that which is part of a unity: symmetrical, equivalent in form, and related

to the center or source through the laws of number. Those earthly phenomena that are beautiful in this way point the human eye toward the Divine eye.

There are many psychological implications in the idea of beauty as proportion. Through a focus on the laws of number, perception becomes transcendent in orientation, moving consciousness away from the phenomenal world. Boethius, for example, congratulated Pythagorus for undertaking the study of music without actually hearing it, "setting aside the judgement of the ears."[23] Augustine wrote that "reason wished to be transported to contemplation of things divine. . . . It longed for beauty which it alone could by itself behold without the eyes of ours, but it was impeded by the senses."[24] Augustine quotes from John, "The Lord has taught the soul of men what they should not love. 'Love not the world' (John 2:15–16)."[25] The human eye, perceiving through the metaphysics of proportion, brings to any situation a normative concept of ideal order. Judgment of beauty becomes objectively valid to the extent that it fits into a scheme of proportion. In other words, judgment comes from without, through a system, not inherently from the phenomenon itself.

The importance given to the idea of a center in the metaphysics of proportion reflects a sense of God as the absolute, the indivisible perfection, and orients consciousness around a single perspective. Proportion subordinates the appearance of multiple particulars to the unity of the source. If there is one source for all phenomena, then all perception becomes organized around a single way of seeing. The metaphysics of proportion, which organizes consciousness around a center, implies a singular way or truth. In this sense, centristic consciousness gives a sense of permanence and eternity. Abstract laws of numbers cannot be destroyed or changed. The singular structure of the way is comforting in the face of the flux of the world.

As well, the imposition of order upon infinitude gives the observer a sense of control. If the Homeric individual was vulnerable to the many revealings of deity, the Pythagorean individual sought to control the unlimited through the utilization of an instrument—number. In speaking of the Pythagorean sense of order, F. M. Cornford writes:

> The infinite variety of equality in sound is reduced to order by the exact and simple law of ratio in quantity. The system so defined still contains the unlimited element in the blank intervals between the notes; but the unlimited is no longer an orderless continuum: it is confined within an order, a kosmos, by the imposition of limit or measure.[26]

Augustine followed the Pythagoreans in their emphasis upon order in the service of certainty.

We have to admit that in number and rhythm, all, without exception and without limit, starting from the single origin of unity, is *complete and secure,* in a structure of equality and similitude and wealth of goodness, cohering from unity onwards in most intimate affection. (Italics mine)[27]

When beauty is seen as measure, particular phenomena are seen as fragmented and become undervalued in themselves. Proportion becomes the mode of perception that is most comfortable because it allows for a sense of control through number and an alignment with the divine.[28] By contrast, when beauty is seen in appearance, the fragment becomes a center in itself. Those phenomena that are skewed and grotesque from a centristic standpoint become rich in inherent value when seen in terms of their appearance.

In summary, although proportion gives rise to a sense of certainty and order, it also favors number over appearance, the unity of numerical system over the inherent value of the particular, and moves consciousness away from an intimate connection with the world. In the next chapter, I shall discuss how proportion as theory becomes literalized into linear perspective, the dominant mode of perception in the modern era.

5
# LINEAR PERSPECTIVE

In Albrecht Dürer's engraving *St. Jerome* the saint is depicted in his study, deeply involved in his scholarly work. The light of *nous* fills the room and centers above and behind the head of the old saint; but the engraving has little to do with the aesthetics of light. Instead, it is linear perspective that organizes the image. The viewer's eye is drawn by slanting lines through a proscenium frame, past the protecting animals, the various objects and pieces of furniture, to focus on the center glow of light. A feeling of centeredness, security, stability, and order pervades the image.

This chapter is historical in nature because it deals with a development in the paradigm of beauty as an inner phenomenon during the Renaissance. The development has to do with the transformation of proportion as a metaphysical system into its literalization as a methodology of representation, namely, linear perspective. In this transformation, the metaphysics of relating parts to a center developed into a method of depicting the natural world. The method, linear perspective, established the correct proportion of the contents of a picture in relation to its center as viewed from a fixed position. Linear perspective, like the concept of proportion on which it is based, reflects a need for control, exactitude of measure, stability, and the security of order.

The medieval mode of understanding the world was through a transcendent consciousness moving from the things of the earth to the wonders of heavenly life. The universe consisted of objects animated and moved by God, referring to him in a unitary, hierarchical matrix. Subject and object alike were merged in the beauty of God's unity.

By contrast, the mark of Renaissance consciousness was that understanding was achieved through the natural world. The intelligible was revealed through the sensible. What had been the determination of the ideal, in terms of a harmonistic metaphysics, became the exploration of nature itself with instruments of measure. It was a time for the gradual discovering of the beauty of the world.[1]

The "discovery of the natural world" and its exploration was pre-

figured by an attitude toward nature exemplified by Francesco Petrarch (1304–47). For Petrarch, nature was not alien and demonic but
a mirror of the soul. In his description of his travail over the landscape
of Mont Ventoux, first through its valleys and then to its peak, there is
a tension between the urge to celebrate nature and the need for a more
purely spiritual communion with God. The two, nature and spirit,
reflect each other in this tension. The Renaissance regard for nature
moved from seeing nature as a direct reflection of divine splendor to
seeing the world as having a separate existence that could be described
from direct empirical observation.

In addition to the sensible world, humanity itself took on the focus
of a consciousness organized around beauty during the Renaissance.[2]
Humanity, as well as God, became creator, and art as the creative
expression of human beings was born. Prior to the Renaissance, art
and craft were considered the same, that which had to do with
"making" or constructing according to the laws of divine form.[3] In the
Renaissance, people were seen as having the power themselves to
create form. The sensible world became the medium through which
the creative force in humanity was at work. Humans were, as Ernst
Cassirer remarks, the "eye and mirror" of the universe, a mirror that
shapes and forms images itself.[4] In fact, the individual could only
arrive at full determinacy by bringing into being his power of creation,
which also served to complete, improve, and refine his world. Humanity, as creator, was the intermediary between God and world, revealing the intelligible in the sensible.

Humanity became the object of creativity. For Petrarch, a person's
life was a process of self-creation, so that the noble human was both
the artist and the work of art. In this way, the notion of personality
was born. Likewise, the human body itself became the ideal subject of
art. Erwin Panofsky writes:

> The theory of proportions achieved an unheard-of prestige in the Renais-
> sance. The proportions of the human body were praised as a visual realiza-
> tion of musical harmony; they were reduced to general arithmetical or
> geometrical principles, . . . [and] they were connected with the various
> classical gods, so that they seemed to be invested with an antiquarian and
> historical, as well as with a mythological and astrological, significance.[5]

Michelangelo revealed the body to be a medium for the expression of
noble sentiment. Botticelli, Raphael, and Titian, influenced by the
Neoplatonic aesthetics of light, painted the human figure in its full
sensuousness. Da Vinci and Dürer, working in the service of measure,
depicted the human form according to an exact scale of proportion.

The discovery of linear perspective was intricately related to the

movement of consciousness from the heavens to the world in several ways. First, the Renaissance was guided by the idea that the micro-cosm reflected the macrocosm and that the earthly world paralleled the heavenly world—"as above, so below." If the heavenly world was an exactly proportionate world, then the world below would be also. As the Renaissance eye moved its focus from heaven to earth, description became more and more exact, and exactness of description came to mean literal measure. The theory of proportion, a system of establish-ing the mathematical relation between the various parts of a whole, became literalized into geometric measurement. God's ideal form and design for things came to be seen as inherent in the laws of geometry. The theoretical space of the mathematician, the infinite space of the theologian, and physical space came to be one and the same. Therefore, mathematics came to be seen as the means for alignment with God. In sum, linear perspective satisfied a spiritual need as well as a need for literalness.

Another contribution to the discovery of linear perspective was the increased interest in the subjective aspect of perception in the late Middle Ages and the Renaissance. Albertus Magnus regarded beauty as a transcendental, objective principle transforming the multiple forms into a unity. For Albertus, "The nature of the beautiful consists in general in a resplendence of form, whether in the daily-ordered parts of material objects or in men or in actions."[6] Albertus's student Thomas Aquinas considered beauty to be objective, but he also consid-ered the emotional or subjective experience as part of the determina-tion as to what is beautiful. For something to be beautiful, pleasure must be aroused in the observer. Aquinas wrote, "We call a thing beautiful when it pleases the eye of the beholder. (Summa Ia, 5, 4)"[7] Likewise, William of Auvergne stressed the subjective experience of pleasure in the perception of beauty. He wrote, "We call a thing visually beautiful when of its own accord it gives pleasure to spec-tators and delight to vision."[8] Man was becoming part of the process of the revealing of the beautiful.

A third precursor to the discovery of linear perspective was the renewed interest in the connection between the metaphysics of light and the physiology of optics.[9] Robert Grosseteste (1168–1253) at-tempted to combine the aesthetics of light and the metaphysics of proportion. He came to see light as being that which is perfectly proportionate.

Light is beautiful in itself, for its nature is simple and all things are light to it. Wherefore it is integrated in the highest degree and most harmoniously proportioned and equal to itself: for beauty is a harmony of proportions.[10]

Much as the point was the most perfect of proportions for Augustine, here, light as "equal to itself" is the most perfect of proportions for Grosseteste. Roger Bacon (1220–92) thought that God's grace "is very clearly illustrated through the multiplication of light." Therefore, to understand the mathematical laws of optics would give insight into the nature of God.[11] John Pecham (1235–92) wrote *Perspectiva communis,* a widely read review of the work of Alhazen, the Arab philosopher of optics. Alhazen combined the Greek mathematical scheme of the visual cone (fig. 5) with a theory of how the eye functions. He thought that rays extended from objects to the eye and were recorded, and he used the system of proportion to explain how the eye could record images of larger objects.

Linear perspective itself was discovered by Filippo Brunelleschi (1374–1446), a Florentine painter and designer who created numerous architectural masterpieces including the dome over the Cathedral of Santa Maria del Fiore. In 1425 Brunelleschi conducted an experiment in which he painted the front of the Florence Baptistery onto a small wooden panel. What made Brunelleschi's technique remarkable was that he painted his image, not by looking at the baptistry itself, but from its image as it was reflected in a small mirror. Reality was depicted not as a world of direct perception involving all of the senses, but as a perceptual field reflected by the geometric exactitude of the mirror. The mirror reflection was taken as a literal replica of the perception of the mind's eye.

*Perspectiva* is a Latin word that means "a view through something." With linear perspective, the "something" is a "transparent window through which we look out onto a section of the visible world."[12] Brunelleschi invented perspective by connecting two premises that follow the model of perception as taking place through a window. The first was that the visual image is produced by straight lines that connect the eye with objects so that the resulting configuration becomes like a pyramid. The eye would form the apex as the horizon would form the base (fig. 1). The second premise was that the size and shape of the objects in the image are determined by the relative position of the rays that make them visible (fig 2). Brunelleschi's revolutionary idea was to conceive of a plane or "window" being interjected between the eye and the horizon. The plane would then allow for the projection of the visual image onto its surface by mathematical calculation of the point where the rays would intersect the plane (fig. 3). If this plane were a painter's canvas, for example, the effect was that "you thought you saw the proper truth and not an image."[13] The perceived "proper truth" became that which was separated from the perceiver by an artificial boundary with the perceiver as subject and the perceived as object.

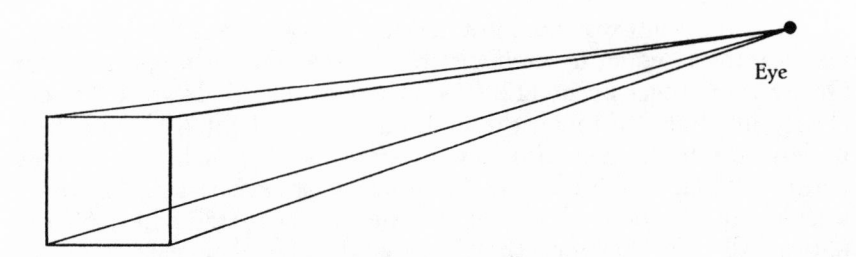

Figure 1. The visual pyramid

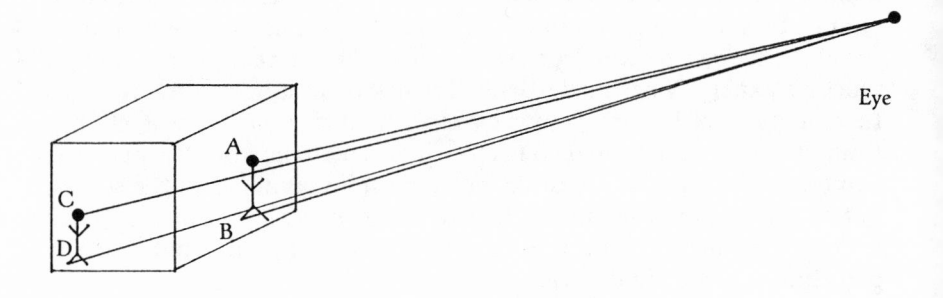

Figure 2. Vision and proportion

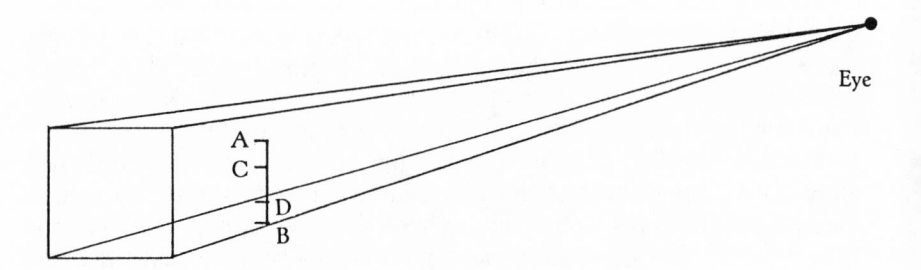

Figure 3. The visual plane of linear perspective

The theory of linear perspective was based upon the assumption that the viewer, through the principles of proportion, could see large objects represented as small and vice versa. The "truth" of an object became not the quality of its form but its measure both in size and in distance from the viewer. Objects would diminish in size as their distance from the beholder increased. The smaller the object on the interposed plane (the painter's canvas), the greater the distance from the viewer. With linear perspective, "reality" was no longer the Platonic ideal image in the soul, but that which was literal, known through sensory perception, and measured as a three-dimensional space composed of objects and interstices.[14]

Brunelleschi's achievement was passed on to the world through the writings of Batista Alberti (1404–72). It was Alberti's dream to take what Brunelleschi had accomplished pragmatically and make it into a science. The science of perspective would allow the painter to achieve correct comparison and proportion through projection of a visual space onto a plane and enable the world to be addressed through geometric properties. Alberti's interest was in providing a standard means for painters to make a pictorial space according to the harmonic laws of geometry and mathematics—a metaphor for the world of order fash-ioned by God. Behind Alberti's dream of perspective as a science was a spiritual ideal or metaphysical "conviction that the beauties of the . . . arts correspond to a moral and spiritual equilibrium of human exis-tence."[15]

There are three major aspects of linear perspective, each with its own set of psychological implications, in which one can see the meta-physics of proportion literalized. First, the inherent relation of the parts to the center of the whole in proportion becomes the geometric method of linear perspective. Second, the center as intelligible source in proportion becomes the literal point of visual focus in linear perspec-tive. Third, the invisible, divine quality of the center in proportion becomes the "vanishing point" of linear perspective.

In regard to the first factor, as in the metaphysics of proportion, the parts of the whole are proportionately arranged in relation to the center; so with perspective this proportion literally can be arranged around the center of the visual frame through mathematical and geometrical means. Linear perspective requires a mental measurement determining the distance of any object from the viewer according to its size. Appearance, or beauty, now cannot be seen without the applica-tion of a grid or lens of mathematical proportion through which to organize vision. The light, directly manifest to sense in the *Phaedrus,* is now filtered through the grid of a conceptual system. (In psychology, these systems are schemes of development, energics, compensation,

typology, or statistics.) With linear perspective the mathematical medium, not the appearance of the thing itself, becomes the ground of
consciousness.

With the second factor, a centristic emphasis from the metaphysics
of proportion is carried over to the method of linear perspective. The
centristic focus of linear perspective is prefigured in the medieval idea
of the centric visual ray. Both Ptolemy of Alexandria and Galen
proposed that rays near the center of the visual cone in which the eye
is the apex were shorter than other rays, hence creating clearer and
more precise impressions of the objects seen (fig. 5). Alhazen incorpo-
rated the idea of a centric ray or *axis visualis* that travels straight
through the vitreous humor to the optic nerve. The rays nearest this
axis elicit the greatest visual acuity to what is in the center of the field
of vision. Again, the center is emphasized as the most important aspect
of the vision.

With its centristic emphasis, linear perspective is a vision that
emphasizes singularity. It implies, in effect, that there is only one true
perspective, the fixed eye of the beholder. The importance of the center
in the metaphysics of proportion and the technique of linear perspective reflects a logocentric philosophical and moral priority in the
Western mind. As Samual Edgerton asserts, "Europeans came more
and more to believe that things planned or seen from a central viewpoint had greater monumentality and moral authority than those
which were not."[16] Singularity of vision, then, takes precedent over
that which is multifaceted.

The third factor in linear perspective is that the lines of the picture
running perpendicular to the picture plane tend to converge toward
one central point at which they ultimately seem to vanish (fig. 4). The
implication is that the lines move toward infinity. The focus of the
picture is organized around this vanishing point, which Alberti called
"the centric point."[17] What is most important about the picture and
about the world it represents is not there, just as in the metaphysics of
proportion the center, as a source to which all the appearing parts
relate, is invisible.

As the center in proportion carries the aspect of divinity, so does the
focus organized around a vanishing point suggest the identification of
the beholder with the incorporeal divine eye of proportion. At the
same time, as vision becomes centralized around a point on the horizon, it becomes horizontal or flat (fig. 4). As perception becomes
flattened, the eye takes precedence as the major organ of perception.
The beholder "looking through a window" looses the bodily origins of
perception. The two opposing centers of perception, the mind's eye of
the beholder, and the divine eye of God reflect each other, giving rise
to a hidden identification of the human mind with divinity (fig. 6). As

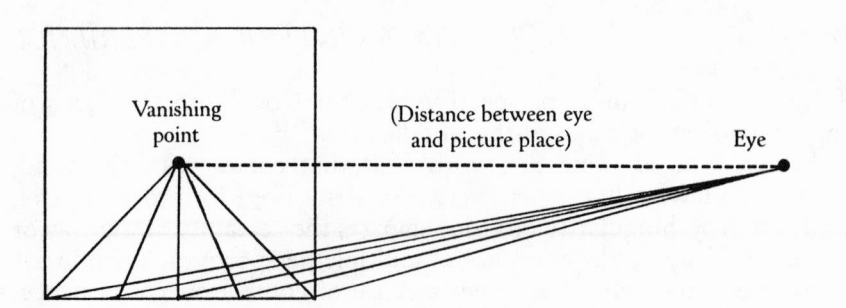

Figure 4.  The vanishing point of linear perspective

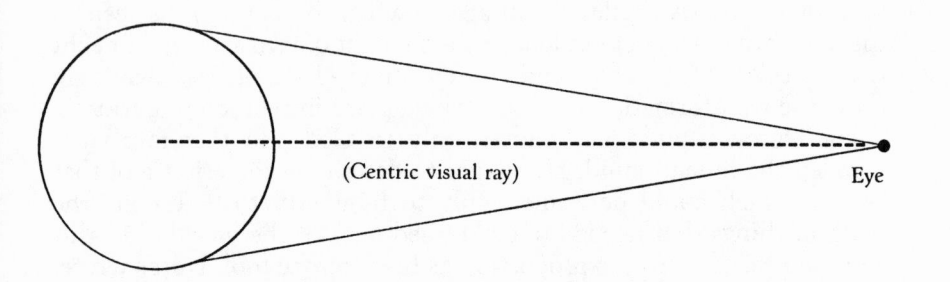

Figure 5.  The centric visual ray

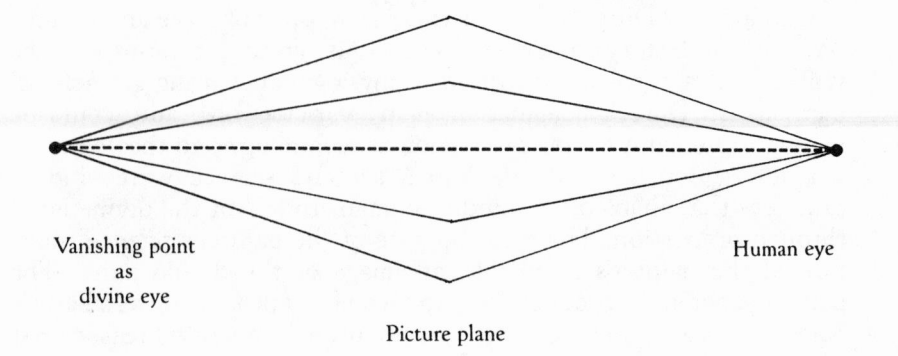

Figure 6.  The detached eye and the divine eye

Edgerton states, linear perspective brought God "into the focus of man, reversing the ethos of the Middle Ages."[18]

In sum, the identification with God that comes with the fixed, centristic view of linear perspective serves a need for order, control, and certainty. Singularity of vision imparts the certainty of the way or the truth, denying the existence of multiple perspectives. With linear perspective, the subject achieves a sense of control over experience. The world becomes something to be manipulated or something that potentially can be used or consumed.

With the invention of linear perspective, what has happened to beauty in the Renaissance? Linear perspective was invented and developed by artists and designers who knew that it varied from the actuality of perceptual experience, denied individual differences, and made straight lines out of natural curves. Yet, the undaunted enthusiasm for perspective reflected an age in which humanity was seen as the mirror of God. A closer look at the thought of two artists, Albrecht Dürer (1472–1528) and Leonardo da Vinci (1452–1519), may help show the transformation that was taking place in relation to beauty.

For Dürer, beauty was known only to God and therefore transcended the human mind. He sought to determine the criteria of that beauty which could be known only to humanity to determine the truth of things that needed to be "pulled out" of the world.[19] In this endeavor he came to use proportion as his ultimate tool. Dürer wrote, "I believe the harmonious things to be the most beautiful ones."[20] Proportion for Dürer, however, was not strictly a matter of measure but something to be extracted through an intuitive synthesizing of the outer and the inner in the artist's mind—"painting out of one's head without aid."[21]

Harmony for Dürer did not always mean forms of grace and symmetry. He saw beauty in skewed, monstrous, grotesque forms, and he worked out a typology of abnormal physiognomies using geometrical methods. In Dürer's imagination, many varieties of beauty could be known to humanity using proportion as technology and theology.

Likewise for Leonardo da Vinci, art and science were kindred processes that enabled the mind of humans to mirror the divine mind through proportion. The divine nature of the painter's science transformed the painter's mind into an image of the divine mind. The painter generated a product using the science of proportion as a base.[22] Science was a second creation of nature brought about by reason. Art was a second creation of nature brought about by imagination. Reason and imagination, then, were different manifestations of the power of humanity to generate form. In other words, for Da Vinci there was no dualistic split between experience (imagination) and mathematics (reason). Each completed itself in the other. Nature became animated

through the imagination, and true imagination could never soar above nature.

The ground of Da Vinci's unified approach to art and science, imagination and reason, was proportion. For Da Vinci, the universe was ordered according to the laws of proportion, which were divine. He insisted upon the possibility of grasping all forms with the literal eye through the mathematics of proportion, a process he held to be the redeeming and ennobling of nature by humanity. Implicit in Da Vinci's idea of replicating God's order through proportion was a sense of humanity's potential to control nature through the creation of form.

In summary, one of the great features of Renaissance thought was the transformation of form (proportion) to function (linear perspective). By transforming consciousness oriented toward substance as given by nature to that which could be designed and constructed through the science of proportion, the Renaissance artist-scientist changed the world from being the product of God's making to being the potential resource of human beings. The invention and elaboration of perspective enabled the drawing of three-dimensional objects to scale. It gave rise to the differentiation of fine and applied art, which eventually led to the development of the descriptive sciences.[23] Now the mind no longer came to rest in the "divine splendor" of natural forms, but it used number in a quest for exactitude of model. Necessity lay, not in light, but in measure. Beauty was seen, not in the appearance of the world, but in the power of proportion. *Pulchritudo* was moving from *bonum* to *verum* and becoming a mathematical principle.

I began this chapter with the "face" of linear perspective, the head of St. Jerome, centered at the vanishing point of Dürer's depiction. At the close of his book, *Psychological Life: From Science to Metaphor,* Robert Romanyshyn presents a photograph of the face of an experimental subject, his head fixed in an electronic apparatus, peering out at the camera. Romanyshyn refers to the face, disturbing in its mechanization, as the "face of modern psychology."[24] I suggest that this face is a part of the progression from Dürer's *St. Jerome* as the face of linear perspective, to modern consciousness. What was meant as a method for painters would become the modern way of knowing the world.

The faces of modern psychology and linear perspective have an even earlier precursor, however, in Plato's myth of men in a cave.

Conceive them as having their legs and necks fettered from childhood, so that they remain in the same spot, able to look forward only, and prevented by the fetters from turning their heads. (*Rep.* VII, 514a)

Plato's sense of the vision of illusion had to do with exactly that fixed,

centristic vision that evolved from his notion of measure and geometry as the means of truth.

The philosopher of science, Thomas Kuhn, wrote that changes in paradigms occur not through the efforts of those seeking new para-digms, but from those seeking to expand the old.[25] The Renaissance saw the fading out of a universe of divine light and its replacement by a universe of human measure. This transition was brought about by a group of men who had the intention of expanding the idea of the universe as God's domain, but they conducted their inquiry through the consciousness of the world as the object of human curiosity. With world as object, humanity becomes god.

In 1625, Galileo, who invented the telescope "from the more recon-dite laws of perspective,"[26] wrote the following passage.

> It appears to me that there is in nature a substance most spiritual, tenuous and rapid, which in diffusing through the universe, penetrates all its parts . . . warms, vivifies and makes fertile all living things, of which power the body of the sun seems to be a principal receptacle. . . . This should be reasonably supposed to be somewhat more than the light we actually see, since it goes through all bodies however dense, as warmth does, invisibly, yet it is conjoined to light as its spirit and power, and concentrates in the Sun whence it issues fortified and more splendid, circulating through the universe, as blood does through the body from the heart. This ought to be, if I may risk a supposition, "the spirit that hovered on the face of the water," the light that was created on the First day, while the Sun was made only on the fourth.[27]

Galileo was later to declare that the ultimate substrate of reality was light itself. Here, he places himself directly in the tradition of truth appearing as the aesthetics of light, and yet his work became a founda-tion of mathematical science based upon conceptual norms. In 1642, Descartes, seeking to establish the existence of God, doubted every-thing except his own thought and moved the universe within the mind of humanity. Kant intended to give the experience of beauty and reasoning equal status as faculties of perception and to establish the former as a link between knowing and morality. The effect of his thought, however, was to lessen the value of beauty as a means to knowledge.

It is in the Renaissance that light begins to die out, the universe starts to turn inward into the mind of human beings, and the world becomes an object to be measured. Out of this mentality, in the Enlightenment of the eighteenth century, aesthetics as the science of taste is born. Beauty becomes subjectivized and subordinate, separated from the fundaments of power, necessity, truth, good, and being, which it inhabits in the paradigm of beauty as appearance.

# 6
# THE SUBJECTIVIZATION OF BEAUTY

Linear perspective in the Renaissance, based upon the metaphysics of proportion of the Middle Ages, transformed perception into the detached, passive registration of "outer" information (object) by the "inner" mind (subject).[1] This form of perception is reflected in the interiorization of consciousness that took place in the Enlightenment beginning with Descartes. Cartesian doubt of the world enabled the human subject to become located at the center of the universe. Humanity became the locus of judgment around which experience and perception were organized. Heidegger comments, "The very way man freely takes a position toward things, the way he finds and feels them to be, in short, his 'taste' becomes the court of judicature over beings."[2] Likewise, Rudolph Gasché writes:

> In giving priority to the human being's determination as a thinking being, self-reflection marks the human being's rise to the rank of a subject. It makes the human being a subjectivity that has its center in itself, a self-consciousness certain of itself. Only the subject that knows itself, and thus finds the center of all certitude in itself, is free.[3]

Truth becomes grounded, not in appearance, but in the self-certainty of the ego—*cogito ergo sum*.

The ground for subjectivism was laid during the Renaissance. Panofsky suggests three characteristics of Renaissance art that presuppose the recognition of subjectivity: the influence of organic movement, the influence of perspective foreshortening, and the regard for the visual impression of the beholder. He states, "The victory of the subjective principle was prepared . . . by the art of the fifteenth century, which affirmed the autonomous mobility of the things represented and the autonomous visual experience of the artist as well as the beholder."[4]

With the turn toward subjectivism in the eighteenth century, beauty was no longer to be an inherent, objective, nonrelational property or principle related to divinity, knowledge, and the good. Instead, beauty came to refer to the capacity of things to evoke the inner experience of pleasure. Beauty was now a subjective experience rather

than an objective principle. The felt response of the subject, not the noumenal appearance of image, was the indispensable and decisive evidence for beauty's existence.

In the eighteenth century, Alexander Baumgarten (1714–62) coined the term "aesthetics" and established it as a separate discipline of investigation. In his book *Meditations* he attempted to argue that poetry involved a particular form of cognition. His second work, *Aesthetica* (1750), was an attempt to generalize this theory, establishing aesthetics as a discipline of knowledge separate from intellect. His aim was to create a science for the "perfection of sensory cognition as such. And this [he considered] beauty."[5] Baumgarten wanted aesthetics to become the arena where states of feeling could be taken as facts to be subjected to measurement.

The central aesthetic investigation of eighteenth-century British aesthetic theory was one of differentiating aesthetic qualities and inquiring into the nature of the experience of the aesthetic—namely, "taste." Jerome Stolnitz considers the notion of "disinterest" as being at the heart of the investigation and as the key notion that brought about the displacement of beauty.[6] As beauty came to be a matter of disinterested perception, it lost its hold on the subjectivist mind. Beauty became relegated to a subcatagory of "aesthetic" and finally to die out altogether.

The subjectivization of beauty can first be seen in one of the earliest eighteenth century British theorists, Lord Shaftesbury. The perception of beauty for Shaftesbury was an interior process occurring through a faculty separate from cognition. Beauty "is immediately perceived by a plain internal sensation."[7] The perception of beauty occurs when the "inward eye" (Shaftesbury's term for a special faculty of aesthetic apprehension) records form.

Shaftesbury associated the aesthetic experience with a kind of morality connected with "disinterest." For Shaftesbury, *interest* was an ethical term designating the material well-being of the private individual. Shaftesbury used *interest* interchangeably with *self-interest*, implying a form of selfish ego concern or a lacking in moral quality. Virtue does not involve anticipation of result or "love of reward."

> As soon as he [the virtuous man] is come to have any affection toward what is morally good, and can like or affect such good for its own sake as good and amiable in itself, then he is in some degree good and virtuous.[8]

Interest in the object for its own sake and interest in the self are opposed, and virtue is associated with the former. Virtue is "no other than the love of order and beauty."[9] Pleasure of the sense is always

"interested" (concerned with self) and hence has nothing to do with virtue or the experience of beauty.

In addition to giving up the notion of reward in the perception of the beautiful, Shaftesbury gives up any sense of action in favor of the "view of contemplation." Seeing now becomes passive, a matter of "shapes, motions, colours and proportions of these latter being pre-sented to our eye."[10] This is opposed to an attitude toward the object based on "eager desires, wishes and hopes," which would evoke action.[11]

Here is the beginning of a theme, the passivity of vision, developed by later eighteenth-century aestheticans, which is a direct carry-over from the invention of linear perspective in the Renaissance. Vision, when detached, becomes a mode of taking a passive stance before the window of the world. (Note the difference in this image of vision as passive in comparison to the images of intense and passionate action in the perception of beauty portrayed in the *Phaedrus* and the *Symposium*.)

In summary, with Shaftesbury, the experience of the beautiful is internalized, made passive, and integrated into a system of morality. On the one hand, there is practical action directed toward an antici-pated goal that will bring about material betterment and is not associ-ated with virtue. On the other hand, there is the realm of disinterest that is the experience of beauty, the passive viewing of the object with no sense of utilizing, possessing, or showing interest toward the object and hence associated with the virtuous. The groundwork is being laid here for (1) the separation of the instrumental or practical from the beautiful, and (2) the association of the perception of the beautiful with a moral order.

Francis Hutcheson (1694–1746) wrote the first modern treatise on aesthetics, "An Inquiry Into the Original of Our Ideas of Beauty and Virtue" (1725), and his thought follows that of Shaftesbury. Like Shaftesbury, Hutcheson designates the perception of beauty as an "internal sense," which unlike other faculties of the mind does not respond to the intellectual and utilitarian features of the world but depends on "uniformity amidst variety."[12] The perception of beauty, then, is a subjective process, referring to the idea raised internally. "Beauty . . . properly denotes the perception of some mind."[13]

The aesthetic vision for Hutcheson, as with Shaftesbury, is a passive vision.

> We find that the mind in such cases is passive and has not power directly to prevent the perception or idea or to vary it at its reception.[14]

> The internal sense is a passive power of receiving ideas of beauty from all objects in which there is uniformity amidst variety.[15]

Hutchinson distinguishes the perception of the beautiful from perception that is sensual, "interested," and associated with knowledge.

> These determinations to be pleased with any forms or ideas which occur to our observation are what the author chooses to call senses, distinguishing them from the powers which commonly go by that name, by calling our power of perceiving the beauty of regularity, order, harmony, an internal sense.[16]

The "senses" from which Hutchinson is distinguishing aesthetic sensing are the senses geared to outside, physical stimuli that Plato regarded as the beginning of the perception of beauty. Hence aesthetic vision, although superior, is divorced from knowledge of the world.

> This superior power of perception is justly called a sense, because of its affinity to the other senses in that the pleasure neither arises from any knowledge of principles, proportions, causes or of the usefulness of the object.[17]

Sensate vision and knowledge, which in the paradigm of beauty as light are seen as being together in the apprehension of the image, are separate in the paradigm of beauty as inner experience. What is aesthetic in one paradigm, apprehended by the senses and embodying truth, is an inner sense that apprehends in an unmotivated manner and has no connection with action, utility, desire, or knowledge in the other paradigm. With the latter, the view of the world that affects the world has nothing to do with beauty.

Joseph Addison also eliminates understanding from the purview of beauty in the *Spectator* papers (1712). Addison located the aesthetic experience in the imagination and opposed it to cognition, the faculty for gaining knowledge. Understanding, in contrast to aesthetic perception, is always "interested" and "serious" because it is devoted to the acquisition of knowledge. Cognition, then, is a purposeful, active pursuit, while the perception of beauty is passive and "innocent."[18]

Addison describes the experience of beauty in passive terms and, in keeping with the tradition of beauty as proportion, associates it with symmetry. "We are struck, we know not how, with the symmetry of anything we see and immediately assent to the beauty of an object."[19] "It is but opening the eye, and the scene enters," Addison wrote.[20] The image of the scene entering the passive mind's eye, again, evokes the window or frame of Renaissance perspective.

Along with disinterest, the notion of the sublime gained prominence during the eighteenth century with the effect of undermining and depotentiating beauty as a force or principle. While Addison relegated beauty to a subcatagory of aesthetics, Edmund Burke made the most forceful presentation for the differentiation of the sublime from the beautiful, taking the sublime as "opposite and contradictory" to beauty.[21] For Burke, the sublime aroused astonishment and terror through its association with vastness, obscurity, magnificence, rugged-ness, infinity, and even light. In a sense, Burke rendered beauty "dead and inoperative."[22]

Burke looked upon the sublime as holding all that is considered impressive and powerful in beauty through the perspective of the paradigm of beauty as light.

> In short, wheresoever we find strength and in what light soever we look upon power, we shall all along observe the sublime.[23]

> To call strength by the name of beauty . . . is surely a strange confusion of ideas.[24]

In contrast to the sublime, beauty's qualities are diminished to those of the small, the smooth, gradual variation, delicacy, and clarity and brightness of color.

Like Milton, Burke associated beauty as weakness with the female sex.

> Observe that part of a beautiful woman where she is perhaps the most beautiful, about the neck and breasts; the smoothness; the softness; the easy and insensible swell; the variety of the surface, which is never for the smallest space the same; the *deceitful* maze, through which the unsteady eye slides giddily, without knowing where to fix, or whither it is carried. (Italics mine)[25]

> The beauty of women is considerably owing to their *weakness,* or delicacy, and is even enhanced by their timidity. (Italics mine)[26]

Here, there is again an implied equation of woman, beauty, ap-pearance, weakness, and deceit.

For Burke, as for the other British aesthetic philosophers, the experi-ence of beauty is passive.

> Beauty is for the greater part, some quality in bodies, acting mechanically upon the human mind by the interaction of the senses.[27]

However, the notion that the perception of beauty can only come
about in a passive frame of mind is most evident in Archibald Alison.
Alison (1790) follows earlier thinkers in excluding any notion of
"interest" from aesthetic consideration including "the useful, the
agreeable, the fitting or the convenient" in objects.[28] But he goes
further in describing a "vacant and unemployed mind" as being that
temper of mind that "suits with" the object.[29] In sum, the perception
of beauty can only be undertaken by a blank or void mind; beauty is
completely left out of the necessity and practicality of everyday life
and the pursuit of knowledge and meaning.

The vision of beauty as separate from everyday life and the pursuit
of knowledge implies that only an elite few can appreciate beauty,
those with "a fine genius or taste," in Hutcheson's words.[30] This view
is available only to the elite because it is superior to the sensate
perception and requires an educated consciousness to raise it above
personal dispositions. Hume, for example, who considered beauty a
"sentiment" and "no quality within things themselves," has a list of
criteria that makes for the "valuable character" who is eligible as a
perceiver of beauty:[31] "strong sense, united to delicate sentiment,
improved by practice, perfected by comparison and cleared of all
prejudice."[32]

Alison's writings toward the end of the eighteenth century brought
the twilight of beauty in the thought of the British aesthetic thinkers.
The failure to define beauty in objective terms gave way to explaining
beauty through associations, and soon the associations led away
from beauty altogether. From a linguistic standpoint, Dugald Stewart
(1810) reached the conclusion that the term beauty refers to no single meaning but only registers the fact that the object has induced a certain experience in the subject. In an age that placed high
priority on utility and control through objective measurement, the
idea of beauty became too abstract and depotentiated to be of further
value.

In summary, in eighteenth century England beauty becomes no
longer an objective phenomenon, a universal principle, that which
awakens and is pursued with active vision, that which is connected
with truth and knowledge, which brings about the best for individual
and community in the most elementary and practical way, and that
which is infinite and most powerful. Instead, beauty is made an
interior experience coming about through the disinterested passivity of
the perceiver, associated with weakness, and divorced from knowledge
and utility. Although it is still connected with morality, beauty now is
something divorced from necessity and available only to an educated
few. In the British mind, beauty, now dispensable, fades away.

The thought of the English aesthetic philosophers was a foundation for the most important work on aesthetics of the eighteenth century, *The Critique of Aesthetic Judgement* (1790) by Immanuel Kant (1724–1804). This was the first modern treatise on aesthetics that was an integral part of a philosophical system, and it marked the shift from one paradigm of beauty to another. Although Kant's intention was to establish the aesthetic experience as the link between the realms of knowing and morality, after this *Critique* beauty disappeared as an objective principle and aesthetics became established as a discipline connected with the criticism of art and separate from epistemology and morality.

Kant's analytic of the aesthetic judgment consists of four "moments" in which he relates "taste" or the estimation of the beautiful to four conditions. The four moments are: (1) Taste is associated with a "disinterested" perception; (2) The beautiful pleases universally; (3) Beauty, itself, is a form of purpose in an object, even though the object itself may have no purpose; (4) The beautiful object is necessarily accompanied by a feeling of delight.

Contrary to the paradigm of light that deemphasizes any subject-object dichotomy and attributes numinous quality to the beautiful object, Kant locates the focal point for the determination of beauty within the subject.

> If we wish to discern whether anything is beautiful or not, we do not refer the representation of it to the Object . . . we refer the representation to the Subject and its feeling of pleasure or displeasure.[33]

Kant is saying that in the determination of beauty, although the object itself has form, our reference is to the subject via the feeling of pleasure or the "feeling of life" that beauty evokes. The subjective experience of something is what makes it beautiful.

> The judgement of taste, therefore, is not a cognitive judgement, and so not logical, but is aesthetic, which means that it is one whose determining ground cannot be other than subjective. . . . This denotes nothing in the object, but is a feeling which the Subject has of itself of the manner in which it is affected by the representation.[34]

The faculty for discriminating feeling, in itself, "contributes nothing to knowledge."[35] The aesthetic perception is thus differentiated from cognition, the act of knowing. Knowledge is gained through concept as opposed to feeling. Kant's intention is to separate the experience of beauty from knowledge so that beauty will have an autonomous basis,

i.e., the feeling of pleasure free from the organizing influence of con-cept. Cognition deprives perception of freedom and, instead, organizes it according to its aims. When beauty is subjective, one might say, the world no longer offers itself forth to be known through direct ap-prehension. Instead, truth is established by perception of the world through the grid of logic and concepts.

Although Kant's intention is to provide equal grounds for subjective feelings of pleasure and objective cognition, the effect is to deprive aesthetic judgment of value as a means for knowledge. Knowledge becomes a matter of reason through concepts. Gadamer states that Kant

> limited the idea of taste to an area in which, as a special principle of judgement, it could claim independent validity—and, by so doing, limited the concept of knowledge to the theoretical and practical use of reason.[36]

Hence, the Kantian subjective vision of aesthetics means the loss of aesthetic understanding as a contribution to knowledge. Gadamer goes on to emphasize the importance of this turn for the human sciences.

> The importance of this cannot be easily overestimated, for what was here surrendered was that element in which literary and historical studies lived, and when they sought to set themselves up systematically under the name of 'human sciences' beside the natural sciences, it was the only possible source of their full self-understanding. Now Kant's transcendental analysis made it impossible to acknowledge the claim to truth of the tradition, to the cultivation and study of which they devoted themselves.[37]

Even though the aesthetic judgment, in itself, can give no informa-tion regarding the world, Kant does allow that aesthetics can lend itself to understanding. The aesthetic judgment is universally commu-nicable through an *a priori,* archetypal, or universal structure of experience that allows for the "free play" of imagination and under-standing.[38] This subjective relationship between imagination and un-derstanding, in Gadamer's words, "is altogether appropriate for knowledge and . . . exhibits the reason for the pleasure in the ob-ject."[39] It is the archetypal nature of beauty, then, that has the power to induce the cognitive faculties to enter into harmonious free play with imagination. Kant wrote:

> The cognitive powers brought into play by this representation are here engaged in a free play, since no definite concept restricts them to a par-ticular rule of cognition. . . . Now a representation, whereby an object is given, involves, in order that it may become a source of cognition at all, imagination for bringing together the manifold of intuition and understand-

ing for the unity of the concept uniting the representations. This state of
free play of the cognitive faculties attending a representation by which an
object is given must admit of universal communication.[40]

Unlike his British forebears, Kant is weaving a tie with cognition
into his tapestry of the aesthetic, a thread I shall discuss further in
relation to his notion of the "ideal of beauty." This tie has a public
quality that Kant refers to as common sense (sensus communis). Kant
asserts that understanding is public in quality in that it contains

> a critical faculty which in its reflective act takes account (a priori) of the
> mode of representation of everyone else, in order, as it were, to weigh its
> judgement with the collective reason of mankind.[41]

Common understanding is linked to aesthetic experience or taste in
that it fosters the abilities (1) to think for oneself, without prejudice;
(2) to think from the standpoint of others, that is, to reflect from a
universal standpoint; and (3) to think consistently. Thus,

> taste can with more justice be called a sensus communis than can sound
> understanding; and . . . the aesthetic, rather than the intellectual judge-
> ment can bear the name of a public sense.[42]

Kant establishes the disinterested nature of the judgment of taste.
He asserts, "The delight which we connect with the representation of
the real existence of an object is called interest."[43] Kant explains that
interest is concerned with delight in the "agreeable" and the "good."
The agreeable is that which "gratifies" (as opposed to "pleases") the
senses or animal appetite, the satisfaction of the "practical" goal. That
which is the good, is so by means of reason and makes itself known
through concept. The good involves the sense of what an object was
meant to be, a concept of its end. Delight in the good is also connected
with interest. Interest, then, involves the "faculty of desire," which
contaminates the experience of the object by rendering the observer in
some way distortive of the form. "All interest presupposes a want, or
calls one forth; and being a ground determining approval, deprives the
judgment on the object of its freedom."[44]

Kant's aim is to make the judgment of beauty absolutely pure in the
sense of free from animal appetite. "Everything turns on the meaning
which I can give to this representation, and not in any factor which
makes me dependent on the real existence of this object."[45] The
judgment made free of desire then bestows upon the observing subject
an "absolute worth."

> Only by what a man does heedless of enjoyment, in complete freedom, and

independently of what he can procure passively from the hand of nature, does he give to his existence, as the real existence of a person, an absolute worth.[46]

For Kant, the object, in and of itself, is diminished in value. The question of the nature of the "real existence" of a thing does not enter into the judgment of its beauty. The judgment of beauty or contemplation is indifferent to the object, therefore free of theoretical or practical concern. "One must not be in the least prepossessed in favour of the real existence of the thing, but must preserve complete indifference."[47]

Robert Zimmerman suggests that Kant's intention in his notion of indifference is to substantiate the aesthetic experience by keeping it pure and uncontaminated. Zimmerman writes that for Kant "the experience of natural beauty is experience of the noumenal world as it filters through the phenomenal world."[48] This experience requires a passivity of mind, i.e., disinterest, in order to allow for the thing in itself to register in its own being upon the observing mind. In this way the perceiving subject is allowed a window into the noumenal world that is otherwise obfiscated by concepts.[49]

Although Zimmerman would seem to be going too far in attributing to Kant the possibility of human experience of the noumenal world, his point does indicate that Kant's sense of beauty allows for a linking of the phenomenal and noumenal worlds. Heidegger's interpretation of Kant clarifies how beauty, through its connection to the good (noumenal), links the soul to its "essential nature."

> The beautiful is what we find honorable and worthy, in the image of our essential nature. It is that upon which we bestow 'unconstrained favor,' as Kant says, and we do so from the very foundations of our essential nature and for its sake.[50]

Heidegger suggests that Kant's sense of "disinterest" is not the common notion of disinterest in which nothing of will is invested.[51] *Interest* comes from the Latin *minihi interest,* meaning something is of importance to me. To take an interest in something suggests wanting to take possession of it or control over it. We see what we are interested in with a view to something else, a goal of our own conscious will. By contrast Kant's sense of the term "disinterest," according to Heidegger, is to

> let what encounters us, purely as it is in itself, come before us in its own stature and worth. We may not take it into account in advance with a view to something else, our goals and intentions, our possible enjoyment and advantage.[52]

In contrast to the agreeable and the good, the judgment of taste is contemplative, mediating, through the experienced feeling of pleasure, between the object and the subject's desire. "It is a judgement which is indifferent as to the existence of an object, and only decides how its character stands with the feeling of pleasure and displeasure."[53] Although Kant's two criteria for disinterest—indifference to the real existence of the object of representation and the elimination of desire—quicken the spirit with a "feeling of life," the Platonic image of the soul, passionately moved by beauty toward the truth of things, has been lost.

Disassociated from "gratification" and "what is esteemed good," the beautiful is "what simply pleases."[54] Kant explains his sense of aesthetic pleasure in the "Analytic of the Sublime": "The pleasure in the beautiful is, on the other hand, neither a pleasure of enjoyment nor of an activity according to law, nor yet one of rationalizing contemplation according to ideas, but rather of mere reflection."[55] Kant's point is that taste is reflective and that there is pleasure, and therefore worth, in reflection. It is through the aesthetic judgment, or beauty, that action in the service of desire is mediated, and the subject can align itself with an underlying moral order as we shall discover.

Although Kant intends a separate but equal status for the faculties of cognition, desire, and feelings of delight, his influence achieves the opposite. If he is understood to separate feeling from connection with the world, that is, detached from "the practical goal" and understanding, feeling becomes relegated to subordinate status. Kant's purpose is to validate perception detached from interest, separated from the subject's desiring; yet, the subject has become the source of determination as to what is important. From the standpoint of the subject, beauty, detached from desire, takes a secondary priority. When the world is seen fully subjectively—i.e., when Kant's "turn to the subject" gets detached from "letting the object be" in "unconstrained favoring"—the world presents itself as available for use or resource through faculties such as cognition and desire that control and manipulate it. A subjectivist world view will, of necessity, deprive beauty of its authority, in that it will demand as authoritative only those answers that are certifiable or empirical.

In short, Kant is intending a superior, autonomous status for the aesthetic in his emphasis on disinterest. He wants the aesthetic experience to be bracketed so that it can be free of personal consideration as a pure experience of the world. Yet, that freedom, by virtue of its detachment from interest in the world, eventually deprives the world of its life and dooms the aesthetic experience to a tangential place in human experience.

For Kant, humans experience through *a priori* universal structures

or archetypal patterns. The *a priori* universal of aesthetic experience is
the potential for the feeling of pleasure induced by the form of the
aesthetic object. I have shown how this *a priori* nature of the aesthetic
experience allows for the free play between imagination and understanding. The universal aspect of the experience of beauty is emphasized in the second moment. A judgment that something is beautiful
involves a claim that the object would be considered beautiful by every
human. This claim to universality cannot be made on a logical, conceptual basis having to do with qualities of the object, but on a
subjective basis.

> For this universality I use the expression *general validity,* which denotes the
> validity of the reference of a representation, not to the cognitive faculties
> but to the feeling of pleasure or displeasure for every Subject.[56]

Beauty is nothing else than a mental state present in the subject, but
this subjective state is universal. In other words, what is objective, i.e.
*a priori,* in regard to beauty is the universal capacity of the human to
experience delight in reflection without reference to action.

A fundamental aspect of Kant's sense of aesthetic judgment is the
notion of finality, specifically what he calls "purposiveness without
purpose." In the third moment, Kant states that we experience beauty
in a thing when we sense in it a covert purposiveness without basing
our judgment on an observation of overt purpose in the object. If we
recognize something as purposeful in itself, we will not consider it
beautiful because it is linked to a desire or interest. There is in the
experience of beauty, however, a sense of a hypothetical, higher purposive will at work.

> An Object, or state of mind, or even an action may although its possibility
> does not necessarily presuppose the representation of an end, be called final
> simply on account of its possibility being only explicable and intelligible for
> us by virtue of an assumption on our part of a fundamental causality
> according to ends; i.e., a will that would have so ordained it according to a
> certain represented rule.[57]

Kant is saying that there is an organic interconnectedness or wholeness in which the object of beauty seems contained. Although beauty
must be divorced from overt purpose, there is a higher purpose or goal
that is sensed in the object. The perception of the relationship of the
part to the universal whole evokes a feeling of pleasure from the
reciprocal harmony it induces in our faculties. The beautiful object
induces harmony, but at the same time, the harmony of our faculties
allows for the perception of the beautiful. The aesthetic experience,

then, is not connected with an immediate, known purpose and there-fore maintains its purity; yet it has the aspect of being part of the purpose of an unknown but surmisable will.

For Kant, beauty is the form of this overlying purpose manifest in the object. He refers to the form as the "ideal of beauty" or the archetype of taste. There can be no objective rule of taste that defines beauty by means of concepts. Instead, the sense of the beautiful comes from

> the highest model, the archetype of taste . . . a mere idea, which each person must beget in his own consciousness, and according to which he must form his estimate of everything that is an Object of taste. . . . Hence this archetype of taste—which rests, indeed, upon reason's indeterminate idea of a maximum, but is not, however, capable of being represented by means of concepts, but only in an individual presentation—may more appropriately be called the ideal of the beautiful.[58]

In bringing in the notion of the "ideal of beauty" Kant again makes a turn in which he distinguishes between "normative" or "free" beauty that is independent of concepts, and the ideal of beauty in which he ties concept back to the experience of beauty. The ideal of beauty involves an interplay of concept with essential or free beauty, hence it is not a pure judgment of taste but is partly intellectual. It is not "free and at large," but fixed by a concept of objective purpose.[59]

> In other words, where an ideal is to have place among the grounds upon which any estimate is formed, then beneath grounds of that kind there must lie some idea of reason according to determinate concepts, by which the end underlying the internal possibility of the object is determined *a priori*.[60]

It is the archetype, then, that brings cognition and feeling, understand-ing and imagination together in playful conjunction through aesthetic judgment.

Gadamer reads Kant to indicate here that form and meaning are one through the ideal of beauty. It is beauty that allows for appearance to carry its own meaning without the need to bring in a conceptual system of interpretation. "There can be no other meaning in this representation than is already expressed in the form and appearance of what is represented."[61] Thus, it is only in the archetype of the ideal of beauty that the intellectualized and interested do not detract from aesthetic pleasure. Instead, the archetypal form brings human vision closer to a direct perception or an immediate knowing, as opposed to the concept that mediates perception.

In the *Critique of Aesthetic Judgement,* Kant sought to validate feeling as a faculty of perception and to give it a privileged position by establishing its universality. He strove to make aesthetic experience, as contemplative, significant by establishing it as a purified experience, free from personal predispositions. It was through aesthetic experience that he linked two seemingly separate areas—knowledge of the world and alignment with divine moral order. On the one hand, aesthetic experience moves humanity closer to a direct experience of the world than cognition would allow, free from the influence of personal disposition and reason. Thus, Kant did not take a purely subjective stance toward aesthetics but saw beauty as linking the objective and the subjective. On the other hand, beauty, for Kant, was the sensual manifestation of the realm of morality toward which it leads the human eye. Through the experience of the beautiful, man would discern nature's purposive order and design, which consists of intelligible properties.

> Now, I say, the beautiful is the symbol of the morally good, and only in this light . . . does it give us pleasure with an attendant claim to the agreement of everyone else, whereupon the mind becomes conscious of a certain ennoblement and elevation above mere sensibility to pleasure from impressions of sense, and also appraises the worth of others on the score of a like maxim of their judgement. This is that *intelligible* to which taste . . . extends its view.[62]

While Kant's characterization of the perception of beauty as a judgment and his initial separation of the aesthetic experience from desire and knowing would make it seem that he belongs squarely within the paradigm of beauty as inner experience, actually, his thought provides a connection back to the paradigm of beauty as light. The archetypal nature of "purposiveness without purpose," the "ideal of beauty," and *sensus communis,* in fact, link the aesthetic experience back to a higher moral order, understanding, and pleasure.

Kant's second movement of integration is not as overt as the first movement of separation, allowing the former an influence that has important psychological implications. First, the subjective emphasis of the experience of beauty places the locus of judgment within the subject, desubstantiating the world of appearance. Second, the separation of beauty from concept, in the face of the rational bias of subjectivism, meant the loss of the tradition of appearance as a contribution to understanding. Third, when the aesthetic experience becomes rarified, that is, separated from everyday concerns of practicality and understanding through the bracketing of personal disposition and conceptualization, it becomes available only to a select few. The transcen-

dental Kantian mind requires an educated consciousness that is elevated or, in Gadamer's words,

> raised to the universal, distancing from the particularity of immediate acceptance or rejection, the acceptance of what does not correspond to one's own expectancy or preference.[63]

Beauty is thus displaced from the core of general experience to the periphery. It becomes located in realms such as art that can only be humanly produced by genius—persons with special talent for an intuitive sensitivity to nature.

Finally, if (contrary to Heidegger) Kant's notion of disinterest is seen as passive, then the opposition between contemplation and action is reinforced. An interpretation of Kant, forgetful of his ideal of beauty, infers no sense of action in the experience of beauty and divorces it from reason. Meaningful relationship with the world then becomes equated with thought and overt action. Perception is forgotten as the basis for thinking and doing. At the same time, because the perception of beauty is seen as passive, aesthetic perception becomes a mere reception of images. Vision as a fixed, passive receiving of images in the subjective mind becomes limited to only one perspective.

* * *

In part 2, I have tried to present the paradigm of beauty as a primarily internal, transcendent phenomenon that stands in opposition to the paradigm of beauty as light. As I attempted to show in part 1, beauty as light emphasizes truth and goodness as lying in the particularity of appearance. Beauty in this paradigm is an autonomous principle, manifesting through appearance. By contrast, the paradigm of beauty as phenomenon of mind emphasizes the unseen universal of which the particular is a part. In this sense, beauty is manifested in systems of number and order.

I have also tried to show how the interiorization of consciousness evokes beauty as proportion, which gives rise to a literalization of perception through a grid, i.e., linear perspective. Linear perspective, in turn, leads to a subjectivized consciousness in which appearance is doubted. As Heidegger and Gasché have given evidence at the beginning of this chapter, subjectivized consciousness places the ego's concerns in a paramount position. The self-certainty of the subject, not the appearance of things, becomes the starting point of knowing. The observing subject becomes forgetful of the interpretive ground of experience. Control, certainty, identification with divine perception, and invulnerability to appearance become the hallmarks of modern consciousness.

In the paradigm of beauty as an internal phenomenon of mind, truth is held to lie in number, beauty becomes a notion of symmetry and wholeness, and aesthetics becomes a separate discipline of perception through feeling. As aesthetics becomes separated from truth, imagination and feeling become estranged from cognition, and the latter takes on the quality of certainty. Human sciences turn to methodology for understanding; beauty becomes literalized in art; educated consciousness becomes necessary for aesthetic perception; creativity becomes a personal matter; and art falls into the domain of genius. Beauty is now depotentiated, no longer associated with truth, utility, action, and an inherent faith in appearance.

PART THREE
# THE RETURN OF AESTHETICS IN CONTEMPORARY PSYCHOLOGY

# IMAGE IN DEPTH PSYCHOLOGY

Hannah Arendt has written that when being and appearance part company, everything is doubted.[1] I left beauty at the end of the eighteenth century suffering from such a split. Perception had become separate from meaning so that, rather than appearance, systems of derived meaning, i.e. the sciences, had become informants of understanding. Reason had become the ground of being: *cogito ergo sum*. At the same time, aesthetics had become a philosophical discipline replacing beauty as the form through which appearance was addressed. Originally linked to the act of perception, aesthetics had now become connected with (a) the modern notion of fine art, and (b) what makes up the aesthetic experience, namely, taste. Beauty as meaning and appearance unified had become split into science and art.[2]

The orientation of the first section was that beauty, when seen psychologically, is the ground of everyday being and knowing. In the final section, I would like to give an account of the recovery of this sense of beauty through depth psychology, focusing particularly on Jung's later thought and psychotherapy as a cultural manifestation of the aesthetic mode. Finally, I attempt to formulate an aesthetic psychology based upon the imaginal psychology of James Hillman.

I would like to introduce the reemergence of beauty in modern depth psychology through two important precursors, Friedrich Nietzsche and William Blake. These thinkers brought two vital aesthetic principles to bear on their work, which later became the ground of aesthetics in depth psychology—the truth of perception unmediated by concepts and the creative nature of human perception.

In approaching Nietzsche, "the artist philosopher," I am following the thought of Alan Megill who resists seeing Nietzsche predominantly as a critic and an analyst and, instead, reads Nietzsche as an aesthetic philosopher.[3] He quotes Nietzsche from *Beyond Good and Evil*, "There are no more phenomena at all, but only a moral interpretation of phenomena."[4] He views Nietzsche as holding that the ground of being is aesthetic and that all choices are ultimately made on aesthetic grounds. Although he indicates how the aesthetic informs the span of Nietzsche's work, I would like to focus briefly on just two

of Nietzsche's essays, *The Birth of Tragedy* and "On Truth and Falsity in the Ultramoral Sense."

In his preface to *The Birth of Tragedy*, Nietzsche wrote that "art rather than ethics, constitutes the essential metaphysical activity of man," and "existence could be justified only in aesthetic terms,"[5] thereby setting up the aesthetic orientation of the main body of the work. The central theme of *The Birth of Tragedy* is the tension between two aesthetic modes as represented in the figures of Apollo and Dionysus. The Apollonian mode is the tendency of the mind to fabricate illusions, while the Dionysian is the less comforting experience of the dark, unknown whole of experience. Apollo is the god of necessary illusions, covering experience with a veil of beauty that protects us from the "terrors and horrors" of existence.[6] Dionysus shatters illusions by opening the way to the immediate experience of the underlying depth of the world. This experience is unbearable, however, necessitating the eternal recurrence of form through illusion to mask it. Apollo represents the power of the psyche to create form through images over and over again, while Dionysus embodies the impetus toward the direct, unmediated experience of the encompassing whole. The two are reconciled in tragedy where Dionysian ecstasy can be experienced through Apollonian form. Meaning is experienced through metaphor, the linking of depth and surface.

In his essay "On Truth and Falsity in the Ultramoral Sense" Nietzsche most clearly develops the idea that the aesthetic experience is an alternative to the mediating influence of concepts. In this view, concepts falsify the reality that they purport to represent. He wrote, "Every [concept] (*Begriff*) originates through equating the unequal."[7] For Nietzsche, the world is made of individual parts, each of which has its own reality, so that "*this* sun, *this* window, *this* table is a truth in itself."[8] Concepts impute to the world something completely foreign to that reality. For example, the insect and the bird perceive a world different from the human world. When a human being is the measure of all things,

> he starts from the error of believing that he has things immediately before him as pure objects. He therefore forgets that the original metaphors of perception are metaphors, and takes them for the things themselves.[9]

When we refer to trees, colors, snow, and flowers, "we think we know something about the things themselves, and yet we only possess metaphors of the things, and these metaphors do not in the least correspond to the original essentials."[10]

Nietzsche's attitude toward the concept is ambivalent. Concepts rob reality of its multiplicity and human experience of its richness and vitality. Truth has become

> [a] mobile army of metaphors, metonymies, anthropomorphisms: in short a sum of human relations which become poetically and rhetorically inten-sified, metamorphosed, adorned, and after long usage seem to a nation fixed, canonic and binding; truths are illusions of which one has forgotten that they *are* illusions; worn-out metaphors which have become powerless to affect the senses.[11]

What is taken for reality is merely "the congelation and coagulation of an original mass of similes and percepts pouring forth as a fiery liquid out of the primal faculty of human fancy."[12] On the other hand, as rational beings, we need concepts, to keep ourselves from being carried away by sudden impressions and sensations.

> [Man] generalizes all these impressions into paler, cooler [concepts], in order to attach to them the ship of his life and actions. Everything which makes man stand out in bold relief against the animal depends on this faculty of volatilising the concrete metaphors into a schema, and therefore resolving a perception into a [concept].[13]

So great is our need for certainty and fixity that only by the fact that we forget ourselves "as . . . artistically creating subject[s]" can we live with "repose, safety and consequence."[14] Thus, the "needy man saves himself through life."[15]

For Nietzsche, the aesthetic as acknowledged illusion stands in opposition to the logic of concepts. Our consciousness is a created consciousness, so that all perception is a matter of fiction. The intel-lect, free from an illusion of truth, is able to transform concepts into aesthetically pleasing illusions. This intellect is no longer ruled by concepts but by intuitions.

> From these intuitions no regular road leads into the land of the spectral schemata, the abstractions; . . . [man] speaks in forbidden metaphors and in order to correspond creatively with the impression of the powerful present intuition at least by destroying and jeering at the old barriers of [con-cepts].[16]

In summary, Nietzsche's philosophy is an aesthetic philosophy, in that the sensuous, structured and restructured metaphorically, makes up the only accessible reality. Nietzsche seeks to abolish the distinction between life and art. The world, as a work of art, is continuously being

created and re-created. Heidegger quotes Nietzsche, "To pick up the scent of what would nearly finish us off if it were to confront us is the flesh, as danger, problem, temptation—this determines even our aesthetic 'yes'. ('That is beautiful is an affirmation.')"[17] For Nietzsche, the beautiful determines us, to the extent that we are claimed in our essence.

Nietzsche's sense of the creative nature of the mind is prefigured not only in Plotinus, who considered seeing and doing as one, but in the Romantic poet William Blake. For Blake, imagination as the creative faculty of the mind is the animating principle of life. The creative imagination is the facility through which humans become active and perceiving beings. For Blake, imagination is life itself, fully creating reality through an interpretive perception of it. "All things exist in the Human Imagination," wrote Blake.[18] In this world we are "Creating Space, Creating Time according to the wonders Divine / Of Human Imagination," allowing the minute particulars of existence to come alive and shine through in our perception.[19] Yet, space and time are but a small aspect of imaginative being. "This world of Imagination is the world of Eternity," existing anterior to time and space.[20] Humanity creates the world into being through the imagination, and humanity as creator is God working through humanity. "The Eternal Body of Man is the Imagination, that is, God himself."[21] "Man is All Imagination. God is Man and exists in us and we in him."[22]

Experience and imagination are inseparable. The world is eternally being made and remade through the imagination, and the totality of imaginative power is what we call "culture." The world becomes not so much what is perceived by a perceiver, but what is created by a creator. In this process, creator and created are one. The world as object, split off from subject, is the fallen world. Imagination is the redeeming act of unification through creation.

For Blake, as for Nietzsche, reality as created evokes art as the paradigmatic mode of being. The product of imagination is most clearly seen in the work of art. As Northrup Frye states, "It is, then, through art that we understand . . . why perception is meaningless without an imaginative ordering of it."[23] This does not mean that only the artist can be redeemed but that all of redeemed life follows the principles of the artistic process of creative imagination.

In Blake's mythopoetics, imagination is personified in the figure of Los, the preeminent creator, in the form of the archetypal smith. The fire of Los's forge reflects Blake's emphasis on imagination as creation or synthesis. Los is the divine artificer, the generative and incubating power from which all life proceeds. He is the builder of the eternal forms of civilization, the architect of the physical world. As such he is

a "Demiourgos," both creator of the universe and a worker for the people, shaping the world in human form.[24]

I have been attempting here to prepare the aesthetic ground of depth psychology, particularly one strain of Jung's work, through two aesthetic thinkers, Nietzsche and Blake. I have shown how two ideas in the paradigm of beauty as appearance reverberate through the work of each: (1) meaning or truth exists in immediate perception of image, as opposed to perception mediated through constructs; (2) the mind is fundamentally artistic in nature, in that the world is created through the imaginative faculty.

The founder of depth psychology and the immediate precursor to Jung was Sigmund Freud, and Jung's orientation toward aesthetics can be viewed in light of Freud. Freud was completely modern in his separation of image from meaning. In *The Interpretation of Dreams* Freud distinguished between the world of waking life and the world of dream life. "What characterizes the waking state is the fact that thought-activity takes place in concepts and not in images."[25] Waking life is characterized by rationality, thoughts, and concepts. Dream life, on the other hand is characterized by an imaginal process. "Dreams, then, think predominantly in visual images."[26] Freud grants the dream a life of its own, "dreams think," but the dream's imagistic expression makes it an inferior mode for him. Freud associates the dream with "regression,"[27] childhood,[28] "psychoneurotic symptoms,"[29] "the development of a psychosis,"[30] and "the archaic."[31] For Freud, the dream image is a mere "facade"[32] with which we should "concern ourselves as little as possible."[33]

The valuable part of dream life for Freud is that part associated with the rationality of waking life, the dream thoughts that lie latent in the unconscious. Freud's theory, based on nineteenth-century laws of mechanics, was that the apparatus of the psyche transformed thoughts stimulated by daily experience into irrational dream images, "pouring the content of a thought into another mould."[34] Experiences from waking life stimulate thoughts that are unacceptable to waking consciousness. These thoughts are transformed through various processes of "dreamwork"—i.e., displacement, condensation, symbolization, and secondary revision—into irrational images that are acceptable to the psychic "censor." In the form of images, latent thoughts achieve representability in dreams. Freud is clear in his intention for dream analysis, that is, to undo the expressions of the night world (images) and turn them into expressions of waking life (thoughts) for the purpose of deriving meaning.

The aim which I have set before myself is to show that dreams are capable

of being interpreted. . . . interpreting a dream implies assigning a 'meaning' to it. . . . and . . . a scientific procedure for interpreting them [dreams] is possible.[35]

The task of the analyst, ever suspicious of the appearing image, is demolishing the ediface of the dream in order to find a latent, rational truth.[36] It is the system of interpretation that is important, not the thing in itself, the dream image. Freud's system of interpretation provides an aggressive movement through the dream as "royal road to the unconscious," exposing the secrets of the night world and restoring the rational grammar of waking life.

While Freud approached image strictly from the stance of rationalist devaluation, Jung had an ambivalent attitude toward aesthetics that is reflected in his personal history as well as his writings.[37] In his youth, Jung's family kept all of its art in a single dark room in one section of the household, an arrangement that kept beauty separated from the mainstream of activity. Jung wrote, "Often I would steal into that dark, sequestered room and sit for hours in front of the pictures, gazing at all this beauty. It was the only beautiful thing I knew." Once as a boy, Jung was with an aunt in an art museum. At closing time the two had to make their way out of the museum past several nude paintings. Jung confesses, "Utterly overwhelmed, I opened my eyes wide, for I had never seen anything so beautiful. I could not look at them long enough." Jung's aunt, however, took a dim view of the spectacle, "crying out, 'Disgusting boy, shut your eyes; disgusting boy, shut your eyes'."[38]

During a critical period of his middle years (1913–18), Jung explored his unconscious life through painting and writing his fantasies. He was addressed from his unconscious by an image of a woman (whom he associated to one of his patients). This "woman within" told Jung that his work was "art." Jung responded by regarding this as a seduction by the *anima* and turned his attention to the figure of the "wise old man" who symbolized meaning. Jung wrote:

> What the anima said seemed to me full of a deep cunning. If I had taken these fantasies of the unconscious as art, they would have carried no more conviction than visual perceptions. . . . I would have felt no moral obligation toward them.[39]

Jung's stance (forgetful of Kant's connection of aesthetic judgment and moral order) was that visual perception was not enough, that true meaning was associated with a moral or religious attitude. In *Psychological Types* (1913–18), Jung criticizes Nietzsche's idea in *The Birth of Tragedy* that the conflict between Dionysus and Apollo is an aesthetic

problem. "The problem then remains stuck in aesthetics—the ugly is also 'beautiful,' even beastliness and evil shine forth enticingly in the false glamour of aesthetic beauty."[40] From this orientation, Jung sees the aesthetic approach as a form of psychological cowardice or laziness in which "the spectator can contemplate at his ease, admiring both its beauty and its ugliness, merely reexperiencing its passions at a safe distance with no danger of becoming involved in them."[41] In "The Transcendent Function" (1916), Jung splits the aesthetic mode from the mode of understanding. He writes, "Aesthetic formulation . . . gives up any idea of discovering a meaning."[42] Here one can see that Jung's position that aesthetics is separated from meaning and action or "real participation" in the world, lies squarely in the paradigm of beauty as an inner state of mind.

Jung's thought on dreams can be shown to hold an ambiguity that parallels Freud's distinction between sleeping and waking consciousness. Jung's ambivalence toward what he referred to as the "nocturnal realm of the psyche,"[43] can be seen in his description of the dream as a "spontaneous self-portrayal, in symbolic form, of the actual situation in the unconscious."[44] "Spontaneous self-portrayal . . . of the actual situation in the unconscious" would imply the display of an image that holds its own meaning. This sense of the revealing nature of the dream would oppose Freud who saw the dream as concealing the actual situation. The revealing is only approximate, however, for it is still in symbolic form requiring interpretation. The unconscious is speaking its own language, and it requires the ability of one with "sense and ingenuity to read the enigmatic message."[45] Jung is making way for an understanding of the dream based upon a system of interpretation of something unknown. What Jung doesn't take into account, is that the meaning of the dream image will depend upon the system of interpretation or attitude toward the unconscious held by the interpreter.[46]

When Jung approaches the dream through a system, he is operating within the theoretical framework of polarities. In this case, the polarity is between conscious and unconscious. Jung is careful to say that conscious and unconscious are not oppositions that are mutually exclusive, but that they have a relationship.[47] Jung poses the concept of compensation as the relation between the two. The dream is a factor generated by the psyche as a display of the unconscious in compensation for a conscious attitude. In other words, manifestations of the unconscious, the dream images, must be regarded with an eye to something else, the conscious attitude of the dreamer.

If we want to interpret a dream correctly, we need a thorough knowledge

of the conscious situation at that moment, because the dream contains its unconscious complement, that is, the material which the conscious situation has constellated in the unconscious.[48]

When I attempted to express this behavior in a formula, the concept of compensation seemed to me the only adequate one, for it alone is capable of summing up all the various ways in which a dream behaves . . . Compensation . . . as the term implies, means balancing and comparing different data or points of view so as to produce an adjustment or a rectification.[49]

Jung's system rests on an ontology of wholeness or balance, not unlike the metaphysics of proportion in the Middle Ages. The dream is a "product of the total psyche," in that it serves to balance one part of the whole with another.[50]

For Jung, the tendency of the psyche is toward an equivalence in energic charge between consciousness and unconsciousness. Here, Jung is on the same ontological ground as Freud in approaching the dream. He has a preconception of a source or meaning (Freud: unconscious thoughts, Jung: totality or balance of the psyche), associates the dream with deviation from or distortion of this norm, and applies a system for bringing about rectification through the active involvement of the analyst. Observation that implies a subject-object split, application of a system, and active intervention all go hand-in-hand in making up the ground that gives priority to concept over image.

Jung's theory of types is another example of a systematic orientation based on a concept of proportion and a subject-object split in vision. After Jung's prolonged period of personal fragmentation (1913–18) in which he came to terms with various aspects of his unconscious life, he addressed himself to the question of what gives rise to different styles of psychological thought. Jung answered this question with a system of typology, which, while ordering the diversity of approaches to psychological life, can also be seen to have provided order for his own psyche.

Jung suggested that there are two primary attitudes toward the world, indicating two characteristic directions of energy flow. One is outward, the extraverted mode, in which psychic life is organized primarily in relation to things, people, and values in the objective world. The other direction is inward toward internal, subjective states, images, and values. Although the attitudes are opposing, they are both present in the personality, and the relative predominance of one over the other determines typology.

Following in the typological tradition of Galen's classical humors, Aristotle's causes, astrology, Kant's faculties of mind, and Schopenhauer's principles of reason, Jung describes four functions of the personality or four typical modes of consciousness through which each personality functions. Thinking and feeling are modes of judging,

thinking according to intellectual formulas, feeling according to values and relationships. Sensation and intuition are modes of perceiving, with sensation oriented toward sensing of objects and intuition concerned with perceiving the relationships or possibilities inherent in any situation.

Each function, in turn, is subject to the primary attitude of the personality. Extraverted thinking deals with objective facts, while introverted thinking is concerned with the development and presentation of ideas originating in the subject. Extraverted feeling is concerned with external standards, while introverted feeling works through values that are subjectively internalized. Extraverted sensation is sensitive to the physical stimuli in the world, while introverted sensation is concerned with a subjective representation of sensate stimuli. Extraverted intuition looks for connections and potentials in the outer world, while introverted intuition finds relationship and potential in internal images and ideas.

Although each of the four functions is potentially available in any personality structure, in fact, they are developed in differing degrees in each person. In addition, the functions are polarized as oppositions so that Jung regarded the two functions on the judging vector, thinking and feeling, to be mutually exclusive—as are those on the perceiving vector. Thus Jung posited that everyone has a dominant function on one pole, the opposite of which is largely unconscious. In addition, the person would have two auxiliary functions on the opposing vector. If my mode of consciousness is primarily thinking, then, according to the system, I will have little access to feeling, and either intuiting or sensing will be secondary modes.

The two attitudes and four functions make up a geometrical structure or grid of personality that is conceptual in style and symmetrical in form, which is analogous to the classical and medieval concept of proportion. Like proportion, the purpose of the typological system is to impose limit on the unlimited, and its four-fold nature implies an all-inclusive quality. Jung wrote:

> The typological system . . . is an attempt . . . to provide an explanatory basis and theoretical framework for the boundless diversity that has hitherto prevailed in the formation of psychological concepts.[51]

A certain trait is considered only in relation to the whole of the system. My thinking cannot be fueled by feeling or my feeling, ordered by ideational life. My sensing of the environment around me cannot take place in conjunction with a simultaneous rush of ideas or a collage of memories, each with its own particular feeling tone. It is the system

of catagorizing that is important, not the peculiar trait or actual experience of the individual. With the number of traits reduced to four, a sense of totality, is gained,[52] but the wealth of diverse traits that make up personality is lost.[53] Fixed in type, the flux of psychic reality created in each moment by the imaginative vision is lost. What is gained is the subjective sense of certainty, of "nailing it down," that comes with an all-inclusive, cross-structure of mathematically predict-able formulas.

In Jung's interpretive approach to dreams and in Jung's typology, there are two modes of dynamic interaction considered in terms of conceptual systems—compensation and opposition. From his systemic stance, Jung regards all of psychic life as being governed by these interactions. Opposition exists in the poles of conscious-unconscious, introversion-extraversion, thinking-feeling, masculine-feminine, inner-outer, individual-collective. These poles of opposites are antagonistic and complementary at the same time, opposing each other but provid-ing what the other lacks, thereby holding a certain tension of psychic energy between them. Jung regards this mechanism as the "self-regu-lating" function of opposites. When one side acquires a relatively inordinate amount of energy, the energy will at some point flow in the opposite direction, a process that Jung terms *enantiodromia*, after Heraclitus.[54] This alternating flow of energy continuously seeks a balance or proportionate midpoint between the two sides.

Jung's structuralist, energic formulations of compensation and op-position, as well as being tied to the metaphysics of proportion, are based on two principles of Newtonian physics—equivalence and en-tropy. Equivalence, the first law of thermodynamics, or the principle of the conservation of energy, states that the total energy involved in a process is always conserved. Applied to psychological life, my waning interest in one aspect of life will show up in increased interest in another apsect. When my involvement in the outer world lessens, the intensity of my inner life increases. The second principle is entropy, the second law of thermodynamics, or the principle of the dissipation of energy. Entropy states that processes proceed from order to disorder, that energy in a system seeks equilibrium. Again, psychologically, if I am one-sided in my interest in the outer world, it will be compensated by a need to become consciously aware of some aspect in my inner life, setting up a continuous striving toward balance between outer and inner awareness.

I am exploring Jung's concepts of compensation and opposition in light of the classical and medieval concept of proportion and Newto-nian physics. The advantage of seeing in this way is that options for action and goal direction on the part of the observer become clear.

Compensation and opposition imply that the medium becomes a goal because it is in alignment with a central harmonizing source. One-sidedness calls for application of the opposite to produce a happy medium.

What is lost in an attitude emphasizing action and clarity of goal is the revealing of significance *within* the display of particulars in any given situation. If I am overly masculine in my perceiving and behaving, for example, what is needed is the influence of a more feminine attitude as antidote. Even if the observer is not inclined toward remedial action, the system has still imposed a preconceived goal or orientation. Two important aspects of actual experience are lost through this imposition. First, once my behavior or attitude is labeled as "masculine," its unique character disappears in the compensatory orientation toward the "feminine." The particular quality of my ability to penetrate, inseminate, or stand firm is lost. Second, the paradox of the fact that opposites contain each other is obfuscated. The feminine nurturing that goes on in male bonding is missed by a perception that sees only through the grid of opposites.

Jung's notion of the self also carries implications as a conceptual model. Jung's sense of the self took many different twists and turns during his career. At different times he identified the self as: the center of the personality, the central organizing principle of the personality, the unity or totality of the psyche, wholeness, the source and the goal of life. Jung's earlier thinking in relation to the self reflects the abstract, centristic orientation of proportion in that the self is the "goal, the attainment of the mid-point of the personality."[55]

> If we picture the conscious mind with the ego as its centre, as being opposed to the unconscious, and if we now add to our mental picture the process of assimilating the unconscious, we can think of this assimilation as a kind of approximation of conscious and unconscious, where the center of the total personality no longer coincides with the ego, but with a point midway between the conscious and the unconscious. This would be the point of new equilibrium, a new centering of the total personality, a virtual centre, which, on account of its focal position between conscious and unconscious, ensures for the personality a new and more solid foundation.[56]

The problem with the concept of the self as a logocentric source is that when experience is perceived in relation to an abstract center, the unique quality and substance of the concrete experience is lost. The experience of my depression or anxiety, although skewed from a transcendent center of personality, is itself a goal, center, world, in short, a unique mode of being.

I have examined Jung's earlier orientation to the psyche in regard to dream interpretation, typology, oppositional dynamics, and the notion of the self, and related this orientation to the classical and medieval metaphysics of proportion, Cartesian philosophy, and Newtonian physics. I have indicated the limitations of this view in relation to an aesthetic vision.[57] However, Jung's later thought reveals a different attitude toward aesthetic vision that moves it into the Neoplatonic paradigm of beauty as appearance and helps to heal the split induced by Cartesian subjectivism.

In regard to the dream again, Jung describes it as a "self-portrait" of an "actual situation." Already there is a move away from Freud in that the dream is not a "facade," but an image of an actual situation. "Self-portrait" would imply an aesthetic approach to the dream image. Jung's just-so attitude toward the dream image from this position is contained in another statement.

> The dream presents an impartial truth. It shows the situation which by law of nature is. It does not say you ought to do this or that nor does it say what is good or bad. It simply shows the dreamer in a situation. Man is so underneath. This is the truth.[58]

More poetically, Jung writes,

> The dream is a little hidden door in the innermost and most secret recesses of the soul, opening into that cosmic night which was psyche long before there was any ego consciousness.[59]

Dream as door is far from dream as royal road. There is no journey of interpretation implied. One can enter or look through a door just as one can enter or see through dream images as they present themselves. An emphasis on image occurs in the article "The Practical Use of Dream Analysis" (1931). "To understand the dream's meaning, I must stick as close as possible to the dream images."[60] In "On the Nature of Dreams" (1945), Jung takes an aesthetic as well as conceptual stance by equating form and meaning. A "psychic situation is something that if it can be formulated, is identical with a definite *meaning*."[61]

When Jung is standing on ground that honors the image, he sees image itself as holding meaning. In his definitive article "On the Nature of the Psyche" (1946), Jung declared, "We may say that the image represents the meaning of the instinct."[62]

> Image and meaning are identical and as the first takes shape, so the latter becomes clear. Actually the pattern needs no interpretation; it portrays its own meaning.[63]

In these passages, image and meaning, appearance and truth are united. No systems of proportion, harmony, oppositions, or compensation are called for in order to elucidate meaning. Appearance itself is all that is necessary when perceived through the aesthetic eye unmediated by concept.

Jung laid the ground for his aesthetic stand in his earlier article "The Transcendent Function" (1916). Here Jung struggled with the split between the opposites of meaning and appearance, corresponding to the split between conscious and unconscious, and eventually saw them as being in a compensatory relationship.

> The ideal case would be if these two aspects could exist side by side or rhythmically succeed each other; that is if there were an alternative of creation and understanding. It hardly seems possible for the one to exist without the other.[64]

Experience wants both shape and meaning; unconscious form wants the light of conscious meaning, while conscious meaning wants the substance of unconscious form.

Jung ultimately came to the idea that the seeming opposites of form and meaning, consciousness and unconsciousness find their union in a symbolic image. (Etymologically, *symbol* means "woven together" or "thrown together.")

> The confrontation of the two positions generates a tension charged with energy and creates a living third thing—not a logical stillbirth in accordance with the principle *tertium non datur* but a movement out of the suspension between opposites.[65]

Jung calls the process of the union of opposites "the transcendent function," a process both giving rise to and effected by the symbolic image. The symbol is, at once, both an expression and "pregnant with meaning." The symbol is the "best and highest expression for something divined but not yet known."[66]

I suggest that underlying Jung's notion of the symbol is the resolution of the problems inherent in a perspective founded upon oppositionalism and compensation. If we see a situation in terms of image, rather than through a dualistic system of energics, we will find the "opposite" already there. Through a contemplative perspective, a uniting image can be seen as existing *in potentia* in any split situation or dualistic dilemma, drawing the personality toward what Jung referred to as "a new level of being, a new situation."[67] It is seeing in terms of image, or what Blake called the "four-fold vision," or what we call imagination, that takes us out of subjective dualism and oppositional seeing to a truly holistic vision.

I believe that Jung was struggling with the inadequacy in thought forms carried over from the eighteenth century—that is, rationalism on the one hand versus aesthetics on the other. Moving out of his mechanistic, energic, systematic, conceptual mode of thinking, Jung began to emphasize the symbolic image in which he found appearance and meaning united. This unity, Jung suggests, makes up the ground of being itself, following those aesthetic thinkers such as Plotinus, Ficino, and Nietzsche, all of whom gave beauty an ontological status.

> My sense impressions . . . are . . . psychic images and these alone constitute my immediate experience for they alone are the immediate objects of my consciousness. ("Basic Postulates of Analytical Psychology," 1931)[68]

> What appears to us as immediate reality consists of carefully processed imagery and . . . we live immediately only in a world of images ("The Real and the Surreal," 1933).[69]

> Psychic existence is the only category of existence of which we have *immediate* knowledge, since nothing can be known unless it first appears as a psychic image. Only psychic existence is immediately verifiable. To the extent that the world does not assume the form of a psychic image, it is virtually nonexistent. ("Psychological Commentary on 'The Tibetan Book of the Great Liberation' " [1939])[70]

> Every psychic process is an image and an "imagining," otherwise no consciousness could exist and the ocurrence would lack phenomenality. ("Foreward to 'Introduction to Zen Bhuddhism'," 1939)[71]

Here Jung moves into the paradigm of beauty as appearance wherein image is not only the "ground" of psyche,"[72] but "image is psyche."[73] "Images are life."[74] All human consciousness, all human "being" is primarily an image-making activity. In this sense, all systemic thinking, be it in terms of types of energy dynamics, is itself imagistic. The grid of typology, the sliding scale of compensation, the symmetry of statis-tical methods are themselves images, but images superimposed onto experience. In sum, Jung's aesthetic attitude can be taken to indicate that all human existence, all consciousness of self and world, occurs through image.

For Jung, as for Plotinus, Blake, and Nietzsche, the process of image-making that grounds all being is an active process. Imagination is the creative activity of the mind, "the direct expression of psychic life . . . in the form of images."[75] In short, "the psyche creates reality every-day."[76] From an aesthetic standpoint, psychology takes on "the wider meaning of the word, a psychological activity of a creative nature, in which creative fantasy is given prior place."[77]

Finally, in Jung, the psychology of beauty as the radiance shining through each form reveals itself not only in his notion of image, but in his sense of the spark of uniqueness in each individual. Remember that beauty in the paradigm of light is the inherent perfection shining through each particular form. This aspect of beauty informs Jung in his notion of individuation, so that it becomes not so much a system of transcendence but a process wherein each individual personality moves toward attaining a unique selfhood, "fulfilling the peculiarity of his nature."[78] The self becomes not so much a central point or central organizing principle or a geometrical form of wholeness, but the unseen goal of becoming "what (one) really is."[79]

In this section, I have tried to show how Jung can be seen to be an aesthetic thinker in his emphasis on the importance of image and his place in the paradigm of beauty as the light of appearance. When seen through the aesthetic position of two modern precursors, Blake and Nietzsche, Jung is acknowledging the fundamental place of image in consciousness and the image-making nature of psychological activity. When Jung turns to image, he returns psychology to soul.

As will be presented in the final chapter, these two aspects of aesthetic psychology are taken up with vigor by Jung's direct descendent in contemporary depth psychology James Hillman. First, however, I would like to attempt an explication of the aesthetic mode as it appears in the most prevalent contemporary form of cultural psychology, psychotherapy.

# BEAUTY AND PSYCHOTHERAPY

Having attempted to establish one strain in Jung's psychology as a response to the modern forgetfulness of beauty, I would like to formu-late a vision of psychotherapy as an aesthetic enterprise in contempo-rary culture. To help in delineating a paradigm for an aesthetically based psychotherapy, I turn to the ancient notions of the *vita con-templativa* and *vita activa*. In her book *The Human Condition* Hannah Arendt describes the contrast between the notions of contemplation and action in the Greek mind. For the Greeks, the life of contemplation or *theoria* meant the consideration of things beyond human effect, the experience of the eternal. Experience that has to do with mortality was considered *vita activa,* the life of action, or life devoted to public-political matters. Action *(praxis)* and speech *(lexis)* were considered part of the *vita activa* and equal in importance. From this standpoint, "finding the right words at the right moment, quite apart from the information or communication they may convey (was) action."[1]

Thought was also considered an aspect of *vita activa* but was secondary to speech. In the modern age, it is difficult to imagine thought and speech as modes of action. It was only during the Middle Ages, however, that *vita activa* came to refer to active engagement with the things of the world. Arendt asserts that Aristotle's second definition of man after *zoon politikon* was *zoon logonekon* ("a living being capable of speech").[2] Arendt differentiates between *logos* (speech) as contrasted with *nous,* the capacity for contemplation, that which could not be rendered in speech.[3] She states that, traditionally, the life of contemplation was regarded as superior to the life of action because it was thought that no work of human hands could equal the physical cosmos made by the divine hand.[4]

Arendt goes on to assert that for the Greeks *vita activa,* speech and action, was a mode of public life through which humans appeared to each other as distinct, unique individuals. "With word and deed we insert ourselves into the human world," writes Arendt.[5] The reve-latory character of speech and action answers the fundamental ques-tion of the identity of the individual in relation to others: "Who are you?" In acting and speaking, people show their unique personal

identities and make their appearance in the world. As a process of appearance, the life of action is an experience of beauty.

Arendt finds that the idea that both deeds and words are human achievements is conceptualized in Aristotle's notion of *energia* (actu-ality). *Energia* signifies activities that do not pursue an end and leave no trace behind, but find their meaning in the performance of the activity itself. This paradoxical idea of the end in itself is similar to the notion of *kalos,* beauty, which has no end other than itself. It is Arendt's contention that it is specifically human to be engaged in something outside of consideration of means and ends.

> Each individual in his unique distinctness, appears and confirms himself in speech and action, and . . . these activities, despite their material futility, possess an enduring quality of their own because they create their own remembrance.[6]

The notion of *theoria,* or the life of contemplation, was expressed by Plato and elaborated by the Neoplatonists, especially Plotinus and Ficino. For Plato, knowing was not problem solving but a form of contemplation. The contemplation of the forms of the universe elicited a kind of bliss or "divine madness." Through contemplation, one grasped the universal in the particular, the divine form in the concrete appearance.

Ficino espoused contemplative life over the life of action. For Ficino, knowing was a matter of intuitive apprehension of eternal values and not a rational endeavor. The road to knowledge was open to anyone who "seriously devote[d] his mind to the pursuit of the true, the good, and the beautiful."[7] The contemplative life for Ficino was a spiritual endeavor, the apprehension of beauty in the divine forms, and, as with Plato, the experience had an ecstatic quality. Of necessity it called for a transcendence of bodily being, a "seeing with the incorporeal eye."[8] But for Ficino, there was also a return to earthly being so that humanity's reason, illuminated by divine light, could be applied to the task of perfecting human life. Ficino wrote of the contemplative expe-rience:

> Entirely at peace, it will perceive through its own perfect transparency the highest impressions in the light of the divine sun. . . . Nor will the mind then gaze as if at painted images, but rather at real objects, of which all other things are images.[9]

Contemplative vision is not a passive but an active process. Arendt states that for the Greeks, contemplation had an inner affinity to

fabrication (*poiesis*) in that the work of the craftsman was thought to be guided by the image or idea.

> In Plato's philosophy, speechless wonder, the beginning and the end of philosophy together with the philosopher's love for the eternal and the craftsman's desire for permanence and immortality, permeate each other until they are almost indistinguishable.[10]

The sense of *poiesis* can also be seen in the *Philebus* (39a) where Plato characterized the workings of soul as two artists, the writer and the painter, making images in the soul, the conjunction of memory and sensation. Likewise, for Ficino the contemplative mode is an active process wherein the imagination produces images. Again, the images are the conjunction of memory (inner) and sensation (outer). Contemplative seeing, then, is an active envisioning of imaging in which a making of images takes place.

To sum up the relationship of *vita activa* and *vita contemplativa* to beauty, *vita activa* essentially is the mode through which the individual makes an appearance, while *vita contemplativa* is the mode through which images are formed through the perception of appearance.

I would suggest that in contemporary life, one place for the appearance of the individual, the revealing of self (or selves) in its unique distinctiveness, is the "talking cure" of psychotherapy. Arendt says that for the Greeks, the space for individual appearance through the active life of deed and word, was the *polis*. The *polis*, in this sense, was more than just the literal city-state. It was the imaginary space between people wherein one revealed oneself, appearing in one's unique being through word and deed. In addition, the *polis* as "organized remembrance" assures the mortal that his or her being shall not be forgotten. In contemporary life, where the public aspect of city life has largely been lost, psychotherapy emerges as the place of appearance through language.

The connection between language and appearance has been made by phenomenological psychology. Bruce Wilshire remarks that the precedent for this aspect of phenomenology lies in Plato's notion that to have the *eidos* or the "look" of an object in speech was better than to have a directly nameable instance of it.[11] The object as present is limited in the ways of its presence, whereas the word simultaneously summons all ways of being given. For Maurice Merleau-Ponty, language is truth as expression. "The spoken is a gesture, and its meaning, a world."[12] Meaning and word are not separate as interior and as exterior, rather, each coconstitutes the other. Language is not a tool to be utilized, a sign pointing to a referent, but it is instead a revealing of being.

"Language [is] no longer a means; it is a manifestation, a revelation of intimate being and of the psychic link which unites us to the world."[13] Expression through language brings meaning to light. Language as expression "confers on what it expresses an existence in itself."[14] In sum, language and thought entwine with each other, meaning presenc-ing through speech. The experience of beauty attains itself through the presentational nature of language.

For Heidegger, it is poetic language, not science, that truly measures the unknown.

> Poetry takes that mysterious measure, to wit, in the face of the sky, therefore it speaks in 'images.' This is why poetic images are imaginings in a distinctive sense: not mere fancies and illusions but imaginings that are visible inclusions of the alien in the sight of the familiar.[15]

Likewise, Gadamer writes, "It is language which really opens up the whole of our attitude to the world, and in this whole of language, appearances find their legitimacy."[16] Following phenomenology, one can see the experience of beauty occurring through the presentational nature of language. In contemporary life, language is revealed as a mode for the reappearance of beauty, as talking becomes cure through psychotherapy.

The image of psychotherapy that I suggest is as a place for ap-pearance in language. Through language, the patient makes his or her own form, and a self (or selves) is revealed. All of the historical and psychic figures that form personality, including the therapist, are put on display. This self-presentation is like a story in which the outcome is unknown. Arendt writes:

> This unpredictability of outcome is closely related to the revelatory charac-ter of action and speech, in which one discloses one's self without ever either knowing himself or being able to calculate beforehand whom he reveals.[17]

I have suggested that the act of revealing is the answering of the question as to who one is; this question is addressed in psychotherapy through the making of images through language. Yet in a sense, it is not the patient who makes the image, but the image that bespeaks itself through the patient. Through image-making in words, the patient becomes witness to the psychic reality of his or her own myth. This form of *vita activa*, the act of revealing of self through language, I suggest is a mode of experience of beauty as appearance.

Contemplative life or *theoria* achieves its contemporary being in psychotherapy through the attitude of the therapist. I have shown that

*theoria* in the Greek and Neoplatonic sense is pure presencing to what is. Gadamer writes:

> Theoria is not to be conceived primarily as an attitude of subjectivity, as a self-determination of the subject consciousness, but in terms of what it is contemplating. Theoria is true sharing, not something active, but something passive (pathos), namely being totally involved in and carried away by what one sees.[18]

This state of "self-forgetfulness" lies in the attitude of the therapist in giving him or herself over in complete attention to the story of the patient. Since the root word of *therapeia* is *therapeuo,* "to wait upon," then the action of therapy is the waiting upon appearance. To "wait upon" also can be considered as inhabiting or dwelling in a world. In Merleau-Ponty's words,

> To see is to enter a universe of beings which *display themselves.* . . . to look at an object is to inhabit it and from this habitation to grasp all things in terms of the aspect which they present to it.[19]

The aesthetic therapist, seeking to "serve" or "wait upon" the soul in all of its manifestations, will unself-consciously sink into a contemplative mode. In the contemplative mode, there is no leader or follower; the therapist becomes a craftsman, at one with the material at hand and the process of the work. The material is the "stuff" of the soul announcing itself or appearing in ways that are odd, unpleasant, alien, grotesque, ugly, and above all painful. These manifestations we call "symptoms" or "psychopathology." *Pathos* means "experience," and symptoms are extreme forms of expression of the experience of soul. Each expression, though deformed and afflicted, is itself a way of life. Each depression, anxiety, phobia, or psychoses is itself a mode of habitation.

What distinguishes the craft of the aesthetic therapist is his or her ability, not only in both giving home to and inhabiting experience, but in seeing the multiple aspects of soul in the experience. Like the psychoanalyst, the aesthetic therapist sees the drama of personal family at play in daily problems. Like the Jungian analyst, the aesthetic therapist sees any of a number of universal myths at work in the everyday situation. In my slips of the tongue, my feeling of inferiority about my enterprises and projects finds a place to live. Because of my anxiety, I am forced to care for myself in a new way. Through my depression, I come to tap, not only my personal history, but a more profound sense of my creative potential. So, the aesthetic therapist sees in the symptom—a way of life, a "complex" from personal life experi-

ence, and a myth. Through his or her interaction with the patient, he or she provides a "container" or "dwelling" for the process.

As I settle in and listen to a wife's complaints about abuse and neglect by her husband, I begin to see the anger and sadness of a girl abandoned and abused by husbands and father and immobilized by fear. The similarity in her relationship to both husband and father bespeaks the persistence of the soul's need to "work through" or fathom this experience. As the early stages of therapy progress, she becomes more and more enlivened as the story of her experience moves from her present husband to her first husband and then to her child-hood. One night she dreams of protecting her daughter from her first husband. Mother and daughter go to a swimming pool where the mother tries several times unsuccessfully to dive into the water, losing confidence each time. Then a giant, angry god appears whom the dreamer identifies as Poseidon. He lifts her high and hurls her to her death in the pool below. As she wakes she feels she has been punished for "thinking I can do things." Marital problems have lead to personal past history and ultimately evoked a universal image that has been governing her life, the angry patriarchal god.

Later in the therapy, I also become part of the image, evoking responses to this god. Together, patient and I embark on a voyage. Like Ulysses, we encounter many storms at the hands of the angry Poseidon, often blown back and forth or off course just when destina-tion is in view. Often, we are without comprehension, having only the reflecting gaze of Athena as guide. Marital problem, personal "com-plex," archetypal dominant, and therapeutic interaction combine into unified images marking our way.

The remainder of this chapter consists of clinical examples of aes-thetic therapy by three Jungian analysts who have courageously pub-lished examples of their work. William Goodheart writes:

> While I am being "supportive" with a woman patient, that is, being "warm" and "nourishing" . . . she is experiencing assaults in her dreams by a penetrating and devouring man. . . . who appears in different guises in her associations; in her outer life, she starts to select such men com-pulsively. We spend hours discussing and amplifying these figures. . . . I "understand." I empathize with her being so victimized, [and] make com-ments on how difficult it must be for her to stand up for herself.
>
> My current view of this situation is that this patient's dreams and associations have been referring directly to me. She has been picking up my semi-conscious attitude toward her through the various interventions based on that attitude . . . My fundamental stance towards this patient, in fact, has been violating her integrity and simultaneously invading and abandoning her. . . . I have been treating her as if she had no integrity, no self.[20]

Just as interventions based solely on theory are seductive, but demean-
ing, so clichéd summaries of sufferings and imaginal wanderings by the
therapist are poor images and tend to diminish the uniqueness of the
patient.

Goodheart emphasizes the need to listen to the patient's images not
only in terms of symptom, complex, and archetype, but in relation to
the interactional field between the analyst and the patient, thereby
holding the exquisitely complex nature of psychic images. He gives an
example of the mercurial play in the interactional field in a case in
which a forceful male patient came in for a first session.[21] The man
was anxious and inquired as to instructions. The therapist suggested
he relate whatever came to mind. The patient spoke of physical and
emotional symptoms and inquired again as to what to do about this
problem. The therapist encouraged the patient to continue. After
talking about positive aspects of his life, the patient asked for permission to smoke. The therapist, who had recently decided not to allow
smoking, impulsively said, "Oh, you want to smoke," and reached into
his desk for an ashtray and gave it to the patient. The patient lit a
cigarette in relief and continued to talk about frequent travels, and
about not trusting his business in the hands of partners, who couldn't
make solid decisions and were anxious at critical times. Further, his
doctors wanted to prescribe valium, which he didn't really want.

"Seeing through" the patient's imagery, that is, seeing in it a similarity with the patient's interrelational situation with the therapist,
Goodheart views the patient as describing the therapeutic interaction.
The therapist's invitation to the patient to explore his inner life, in
contrast to a concrete, problem-solving approach, evoked an image of
partners. But after the therapist acquiesced to his own anxiety and
indulged the patient's request for concrete gratification, the patient
comments that his "partner," in this case, the therapist, couldn't be
trusted to make solid decisions. In fact, the "doctor," i.e., the therapist,
resorted to colluding with the patient in the use of a chemical, anti-
anxiety agent, i.e., cigarettes. In this case, the vigilant therapist, perceiving with a metaphorical vision, would see his own place in the
patient's imagery, reflecting the complexity of seemingly ordinary re-
porting. This is not causal reasoning or reductive analysis, interpreting
the manifest in terms of the latent, but it is rather "seeing through" from
an ontological position that includes external reality in psychic reality.

Sally Parks gives other examples of this kind of therapeutic seeing.[22]
A client who previously had been quite contained and refined in her
presentation, left a session expressing anger for the first time, directing
it at the therapist. At the beginning of the next session the patient did
not allude to this anger but instead reported an incident in which her

daughter had been given emergency treatment by a doctor with insen-
sitivity and impersonality. In addition, the daughter had been wrongly
prescribed a medication on a previous occasion by the same doctor.
The therapist realized that the patient, in effect, was telling her that
she had treated her insensitively and given a "wrong prescription."
The therapist then realized that two sessions previously she had interpreted a dream with a particular lack of empathy. The therapist
suggested that the patient's report might well be an image of her
experience of the therapist. The patient denied any similarity but went
on to talk of the similarity between the doctor and her mother, whom
she had portrayed as insensitive and unempathic. At that point, the
patient remembered an exceptional occasion when the mother had
been affectedly empathic. The therapist saw this as a change in the
internal image of her mother brought about by the change in her
experience of the therapist.

In another example, Parks relates how a therapeutic interpretation
based on theory produced associations in a patient suggesting that the
interpretation had little relevance for her personally. The patient then
described images of herself as a slow learner in a swimming class. The
therapist saw this as an image of the therapy situation where the
patient experienced herself as inadequate.

Another example of the aesthetic mode in therapy including images
of patient-therapist interaction is provided by Nathan Schwartz-Salant.[23] I would like to explore Schwartz-Salant's work in particular
detail because it clearly describes how the images perceived by the
therapist can hold meaning on an interactional, historical, and universal level and, in their complexity, contain healing power.

Schwartz-Salant states in his article "On the Subtle-Body Concept
in Clinical Practice" that it is often the "direct-discovery" or direct
perception of unconscious factors rather than interpretation that bene-
fits the analytic process.[24] He suggests that our feelings and actions in
regard to relationship are organized around unconscious images or
forms. In the analytical setting, an image emerges between patient and
analyst, a manifestation of the "subtle body." The subtle body is a
realm between mind and matter that manifests itself in imaginal forms.
The image in which Schwartz-Salant is particularly interested is that
of heterosexual coupling as elicited by the bipolar field of analyst and
patient.

An unconscious couple is sometimes discovered in memories related to
parental interactions. Often these were tortuous events, which became a
familial way of life. A child may have tried to protect one parent from the

other, or himself or herself from both. Such experiences formed a continual traumatic process which then became an unconscious model for life.[25]

The structure with which he is concerned is the *coniunctio* or the process of alternating separation and fusion of the imaginal couple following the vicissitudes of the patient-analyst relationship.

The notion of the subtle body brings Schwartz-Salant's attention to seeing rather than doing. He is more interested in the details of the vision of the unconscious situation than in interpreting vis-à-vis a theory, such as psychological development. In addition, Schwartz-Salant finds the images of the couple deepened by the archetypal amplification given to them by alchemical images. In other words, the images of *coniunctio* are given universal validity by images in religion, myth, alchemy, and other imaginal models of psychic processes. Finally, Schwartz-Salant finds the image itself to be the healer in the therapeutic process.

> The primary source of healing lies in the process the analyst and patient have lived through. . . . The imaginal, archetypal couple, the *coniunctio,* is the source of healing that can be introjected by the patient and, it should be added, by the therapist as well.[26]

In his first case presentation, Schwartz-Salant describes finding himself tending toward withdrawal and depression in the face of what seems to be his patient's, Kate, manic style. As he stays with his feelings he is able to identify the two poles of mania and depression playing in the subliminal field between himself and her. He refrains from assigning a causal source through interpretation, but chooses rather to *see* the two aspects emerge from their prior fused state.

> Metaphorically, I attempt to make imaginal contact with her by seeing, in William Blake's sense, *through* my eyes rather than with them. This process involves a sacrifice of clarity, an act of lowering the consciousness gained in differentiating the field into the opposites manic/depressive. . . . This is a process of becoming less conscious and less active, in a sense dumb.[27]

As Schwartz-Salant describes it, when he confines himself to the imaginal seeing of his patient, himself, and the play of mania and depression between them, he is able to perceive Kate's terror; but he says nothing. His emphasis on just seeing and restraining himself from an overt intervention enables Kate to see her own terror. She says, "I've been avoiding you; I have been terrified of making contact. I am scared of sexual feelings and the vulnerability they bring."[28] The

therapist's action here is an act of integrating the moment through "the act of *seeing*, of looking and waiting for something to appear, for some kind of *sight* to emerge."[29] This act is an aesthetic enterprise. "A perception of beauty lingers, a beauty of wholeness and its mystery that would have been destroyed by 'making the unconscious conscious.' "[30]

In a second case presentation, the patient, Nora, begins a session by yawning and presenting a check for less than the correct amount. During the session, she talks about her newly found sense of authoritativeness. Schwartz-Salent describes his experience of seeing through her new sense of herself, "I began to *see* a pocket of contempt."[31] Again, he emphasizes seeing instead of overt doing through interpretation, sacrificing ego certainty for an imaginal sense that was more faithful to the actual situation.

> The clarity of contents and process, especially developmental considerations, become a background issue; the more hazy and imaginal processes become the foreground. . . . It was not that more 'shadow integration' was necessary, nor was any interpretation of the transference or countertransference useful. Rather, what proved to be important was an imaginal process.[32]

Because he kept his "imaginal eye" on his patient's "pocket" of contempt for him, Schwartz-Salant's patient was eventually able to see it as well. She then dreamed a dream with an image of a double-headed, crowned eagle, a universal image of a unification of the psychic split in her emotions.

In his third case presentation, more overt images of the imaginal couple appear in the analyst/patient configuration. Paula had a history of acting out sexually with previous analysts. Schwartz-Salant describes the sexual energy that was evoked in the "subtle body" between them as "a kind of texturing of space in which we both seem to be inside something that is also between us."[33] In this space, Schwartz-Salant is able to perceive an image of an imaginal couple in which the male is acting in a sexually sadistic way toward the female.

> There are two "objects": a couple made up of me and the patient, and the imaginal couple whose presence can be sensed and their form imaginally *seen* in the space between us.[34]

When the analyst takes this contemplative stance, the patient is able to see the image of the repressed abuse her father administered to her and the accompanying feelings of rage.

Eventually during the course of treatment, the imaginal couple

evoked by the patient/analyst relationship is seen by both in an act of intercourse.

> Somthing new began to occur. We could both imaginally *see* and *experience* a couple, but it was very different from the previous one. The couple seemed to hover in the space between us, engaged in a tantric-like sexual embrace that determined the energy field we experienced.[35]

This *coniunctio* is an image of transformation and union, a display of the healing that had taken place through the analytical relationship. Schwartz-Salant reports that after the image of sexual union appeared, sexuality no longer dominated their relationship. Instead, the therapeutic relationship became centered around a different bodily metaphor—the heart.

> It was clear that an answer had been given to her question: "How do the energies change?" They change by working their own transformation, by opening the heart. As always in the *coniunctio* experience, but especially in a heart-centered vision, both people feel a kind of linking of their bodies. Flesh and blood feels exchanged in this subtle-body experience.[36]

Karl Kerenyi wrote that *theoria* is "to look god in the face."[37] The contemplative mode for the therapist is being present to the appearance of the ultimate powers and the inexhaustible being of things as they present themselves in the therapeutic moment—manifestations of the patient's conscious and unconscious life, manifestations of the therapist's own conscious and unconscious life, and the interaction of the conscious and unconscious life of therapist and patient. It is this vigilant attitude toward patient, self, and the space between, the complete presencing to the psychological powers at play, the seeing that is an entering into and inhabiting of another world that is the essential stance of the psychotherapist.

# 9
# TOWARD A PSYCHOLOGY OF APPEARANCE

Expanding the idea of depth psychology and psychotherapy as arenas for the return of beauty in modern consciousness, I would like to conclude with a short explication of the aesthetic attitude as a ground for psychology. I believe that the recovery of beauty is important as a movement toward healing the wound in the modern psyche caused by the separation of appearance and being. The symptom of this separa-tion, Cartesian doubt of the world, reveals the anxiety of con-sciousness without a home. Without a sense of dwelling, the modern mind is constantly on a journey, incessantly focused upon the horizon in search of meaning. The purpose of the recovery would be to bring consciousness back to dwelling. When meaning is seen in appearance at hand, then beauty provides a habitat for consciousness.

Likewise, in beauty psychology finds its home. Without an aesthetic foundation, psychology loses its ground and becomes an endeavor of perpetual journey: research chases its own tail in never-ending circles of statistical analysis; psychoanalysis becomes interminable as a therapeutic endeavor, striving incessantly to recover hidden meaning; and the psychologist can never become im-pressed, in-formed, or touched by necessity outside of his or her preconceptions. The aes-thetic attitude is important for psychology because, without it, the ego remains the seat of judgment. It is the scientist's aesthetic sense, not the knowledge of scientific method, that leads to discovery. Therefore, it is toward a vision of psychology as an aesthetic enterprise that I will orient this final chapter.

An aesthetic psychology is a way of coming to know soul through seeing as opposed to doing. Gaston Bachelard writes, "Beauty works actively on the perceptible. Beauty gives relief to the contemplated world and is an elevation in the dignity of seeing at the same time."[1] Plato showed that truth lies in revealing, *aletheia,* and that *alethia* is the essential element in beauty. Beauty is the way that truth reveals itself. The Greek word *eidenai,* "to know," is a derivative of *eiden,* "to see." One sees first; then one knows.

The aesthetic psychologist acts as a reflector of the image. His or her research question becomes not "What caused this?" but "How does this appear?" In the *Phaedrus* (255d), Plato characterizes the loved one of the lover as a "mirror in which he beholds himself." James Hillman writes, "Reflection refers to the very aesthetic quality of any event, its sheen and shape, the luster of its skin. Event itself is image."[2] So, the aesthetic psychologist will regard any individual presentation of thing, event, experience, or personality as a reflection of its own unique light. Likewise, the aesthetic therapist becomes like a river, carrying the burden of the patient's pain, while reflecting back its image. This counterreflection does not have the purity of the exact replica that a mirror reflects. Instead, it is a shimmering image, deepened through the analyst's own consciousness and the revealing of the underlying myth.

The aesthetic attitude would be the kind of attitude that Plato says is at the beginning of all philosophy—the shocked wonder (*thar-mazein*) at the miracle of being.[3] In the same way that Plato used earthly beauty as the beginning of the philosophical ascent, the aes-thetic psychologist would always start by valuing what is given, the material with which he or she is working. The therapist starts with the symptom—the depression, the fear, the physiological malady, the feel-ing of dis-ease—and sees a god at work in this initial "stuff." Jung wrote,

> The difficulties of our psychotherapeutic work teach us to take truth, goodness, and beauty where we find them. They are not always found where we look for them: often they are hidden in the dirt or are in the keeping of the dragon. *In stercore invenitur* (it is found in filth) runs an alchemical dictum.[4]

The aesthetic psychologist is small minded, noticing closely the detail of the appearance of things. He or she values and cares for these appearances—the discarded, depleted, abandoned, split-off, frag-mented, rustic, horrible, vulgar, repulsive, obscene, and perverse—as themselves being the dispossessed centers of a certain beauty.

An attitude of shocked wonder takes away the literal eye as the primary organ of sense. "I see it feelingly," says the blinded, but wisened, Gloucester. R. B. Onians finds a connection between *aisthesis* and breathing.[5] The organ of seeing aesthetically would be not so much the literal eye, but the nose of intuition. The nose knows, James Joyce continually tells us. Joyce's word for nasal, poetic knowing is "sound dance," a psychological and mythical knowing. In his novel, *Finnegan's Wake,* he writes:

In the buginning is the woid, in the muddle is the sounddance and

thereinofter you're in the unbewised again, vund vulsyvolsy. You talker dunsker's brogue men we our souls speech obstruct hostery. . . . Talk of Paddy barke's echo! Kick nuck, Knockcastle! Muck! And you'll nose it, O you'll nose it, without warnword from we.[6]

Following David Miller's analysis, the nose's way of knowing occurs when we are in the "muddle" of experience, when some "void" happens to us. We know from a word that will "bug" us and lead us to a language of soul that we "obstruct."[7]

Hillman associates aesthetic perception with the heart, the organ to which Aristotle thought passages led from all the sense organs.

Beauty means the forming of what is presented, that which is breathed in *aisthesis,* and by which the value of each particular thing strikes the heart, the organ of aesthetic perception, where judgements are heartfelt re- sponses.[8]

As seer, the aesthetic psychologist makes *aisthesis* more than just sensate perception. He or she sees both appearance and meaning combined in image. Following Gadamer, the aesthetic psychologist approaches understanding as an encounter with something that pre- sents itself or shines forth as truth. (The etymology of "conscious" is "to know with.") This encounter has the character of simultaneity so that experience holds truth. In Gadamer's sense, all understanding follows the experience of art. The aesthetic psychologist does not feel impelled to further relate what he or she sees to a universal, a known experience, an intended purpose, or a rational system for deriving meaning, all of which involve a forgotten interpretive framework. The aesthetic psychologist sees no referent in the image beyond itself, nor needs to find meaning other than in the reality that is directly given.

The hallmark of aesthetic vision, then, is "staying with" or "dwell- ing."[9] The aesthetic psychologist is able, in Gadamer's words, "to experience from the 'occasion' of its coming-to-presentation, a con- tinued determination of its significance."[10] In therapy, as Jung tells us, there is no goal beyond the work itself. The aesthetic vision closes the gap between goal, final cause, *telos,* "that for the sake of which," and appearance. Aesthetic knowing is immediate knowing. In this sense, the distinction between sensuous and suprasensuous is deconstructed so that meaning and appearance become one. The sensuous is then seen as reality proper in that what can be perceived by the senses, the *aistheton,* lets the non-sensuous, the *noeton,* shine through. The image at hand holds both concrete physicality and invisible significance.[11]

The aesthetic vision is a paradoxical vision that contains a unity and a plurality of perspectives. Hillman asserts that the aesthetic vision

brings together the material, spiritual, and psychic—the concrete sensation, spiritual meaning, and the psychic image.[12] In other words, for
Hillman, the aesthetic vision, which experiences soul in matter, runs
counter to the spiritual, which seeks to extract spirit or singularity of
meaning from matter. If being is *Schein* in the sense of shining through,
then reality would have many perspectives. Aesthetic vision would be,
as Plato said, the sight of "the same thing at once as one and as an
indefinite plurality (*Rep.* 525a)." In the *Philebus* (16c), Socrates relates
how the "men of old" declared that all things consist of one and a
many and have in their nature a conjunction of limit and unlimited-
ness. Jung considered this paradox in terms of the single light of the
source (*numen*) and the many luminosities of soul, "the fiery sparks of
the world soul."[13] In sum, the aesthetic vision holds ambiguity, paradox, and multiple meaning.

The aesthetic attitude grants to beauty the ontological status it held
with Plato, Plotinus, and Ficino, as well as an epistemological status.
The aesthetic psychologist understands being as self-presentation and
sees understanding as an event in which he participates through his
very being. According to Hillman,

> Beauty is an epistemological necessity; it is the way in which the Gods
> touch our senses, reach the heart and attract us into life.
>
>     As well, beauty is an ontological necessity grounding the sensate par-
> ticularity of the world.[14]

Henri Corbin refers to beauty as the "supreme theophany, divine self-
revelation."[15] The Neoplatonists regard beauty as simply manifestation, the display of phenomena, appearances as such, created as they
are, in the forms that they are given. If all creatures, things, and events
exist to be perceived, the aesthetic psychologist would see beauty as
the shining through of the suprasensuous in the simple bare facts—the
raw data. To paraphrase Heidegger, things thing, occurrences occur,
worlds world because they are beautiful.

James Hillman declares finally that beauty and soul are inherently
connected. "Soul is born in beauty, and feeds on beauty and requires
beauty for its life."[16] The aesthetic psychologist is of necessity a
psychological aesthete because he or she sees the soul's essence as
beauty. When psyche appears, then beauty is revealed; where the
voluptuous eye is attracted, there is soul.

# NOTES

## INTRODUCTION

1. Ronald Schenk, "Bare Bones: The Aesthetics of Arthritis," in *The Body in Analysis*, ed. Nathan Schwartz-Salant and Murray Stein (Wilmette, Illinois: Chiron Publications, 1986).
2. Hannah Arendt, *The Life of the Mind: Thinking* (New York: Harcourt Brace Jovanovich, 1977), 19.
3. Richard Onians, *The Origins of European Thought* (New York: Arno Press, 1973), 74–75.
4. Zeno used the term *aisthesis* explicitly to mean "of the soul." See *A Greek-English Lexicon*, comp. Henry L. Liddel and Robert Scott (Oxford: Clarendon Press, 1925), 42.
5. Ibid., 870.
6. Hans Georg Gadamer, *Truth and Method* (New York: Crossroad, 1982), 434. Aristotle equates the beautiful with that which is free from the necessities of life and from use (*Politics* 1333 a 30 and 1332 b 32). He delineates three ways of organizing life that people might choose around the notion of beauty. First, is the life of bodily pleasure in which beauty is consumed. Second, is the life devoted to the *polis* where excellence produces beautiful deeds. Finally, there is the life of the philosopher, which is devoted to things of eternal beauty. See Hannah Arendt, *The Human Condition* (Chicago: The University of Chicago Press, 1958), 13.
7. *A New English Dictionary on Historical Principles*, ed., James A. H. Murray (Oxford: Clarendon Press, 1888), 744.
8. Martin Heidegger, "Poetically Man Dwells," in *Poetry, Language, Thought*, trans. Albert Hofstadter (New York: Harper and Row, 1971), 225–26.
9. Martin Heidegger, "The Origin of the Work of Art," in *Poetry, Language and Thought*, 81.
10. Gadamer, *Truth and Method*, 443–44.
11. Edward Casey, "Toward an Archetypal Imagination," in *Spring, 1974* (New York: Spring Publishing Company, 1974).
12. See Alphonso Lingis, "Khajuraho," in *Excesses: Culture and Eros* (Albany: State University of New York Press, 1983) for a phenomenological description of the erotic vision.
13. See James Hillman, "Natural Beauty Without Nature," in *Spring, 1985* (Dallas: Spring Publishing Company, 1985).
14. Kathleen Raine, "The Use of the Beautiful," in *Defending Ancient Springs* (West Stockbridge, Mass.: Lindesfarne Press, 1967), 167–68.
15. For this reason, modern art criticism often equates the word *beauty* with *inexpressive!* See Jerome Stolnitz, "Beauty: Some Stages in the History of an Idea," *Journal of the History of Ideas* 22, no. 2 (1961): 185.
16. Raine, "The Use of the Beautiful," 167.
17. Ranier Rilke, "The First Elegy," in *Duino Elegies*, trans. J. B. Leishman and Stephen Spender (New York: W. W. Norton, 1967).
18. *Enneads* 1.6.7. References to Plotinus's work are from *Plotinus: The Enneads*, trans. Stephen MacKenna (London: Faber and Faber, 1956).
19. See James Hillman, *Dream and the Underworld* (New York: Harper and Row, 1979).

20. Neil Micklem, "The Intolerable Image, The Mythic Background of Psychosis," in *Spring, 1979* (Dallas: Spring Publications, 1979).

21. The myths of Prometheus stealing fire, the punishing Judeo-Christian God bringing about the end of the world, and the Teutonic wolf-god Fafnir swallowing the sun all provide background and depth to the contemporary myth of the bomb.

22. Micklem, *The Intolerable Image,* 8.

23. Rafael Lopez-Pedraza, "Moon-Madness-Titanic Love, A Meeting of Pathology and Poetry," in *Images of the Untouched,* ed. Joanne Stroud and Gail Thomas (Dallas: Spring Publications, 1982).

24. Hannah Arendt's *Eichmann in Jerusalem: A Report on the Banality of Evil* (New York: Penguin Books, 1977) presents the idea that the absence of thought itself is what underlies evil. I am suggesting that evil may lie in the poverty of image.

25. Plato, *Symposium,* trans. Michael Joyce, in *The Collected Dialogues of Plato,* ed. Edith Hamilton and Huntington Cairnes (Princeton: Princeton University Press, 1961).

26. As quoted by Paul Kristeller in *The Philosophy of Marsilio Ficino,* trans. Virginia Connant (Gloucster, Mass.: Peter Smith, 1964), 60.

27. As quoted by Ginette Paris in *Pagan Meditations* (Dallas: Spring, 1987), 157.

## CHAPTER 1. APHRODITE

1. *The Iliad of Homer,* 3, 156–57, trans. Richmond Lattimore (Chicago: The University of Chicago Press, 1951)

2. Gadamer, *Truth and Method,* 437.

3. The appropriateness of personifying as a psychological mode is elaborated by James Hillman in *Re-Visioning Psychology* (New York: Harper and Row, 1975), 14–15. Hillman sees personifying as an act of ensouling, of giving form to configurations of the soul in a manner proper to the soul. He regards personifying as a way of "knowing through the heart." Hillman writes, "Personifying not only aids discrimination; it also offers another avenue of loving, of imagining things in a personal form so that we can find access to them with out hearts. . . . Personifying is thus a way of knowing, especially knowing what is invisible, hidden in the heart."

4. "To Aphrodite," in *The Homeric Hymns,* trans. Thelma Sargent (New York: W. W. Norton, 1973), no. 6: 54.

5. Hesiod, "The Works and Days" in *Hesiod,* trans. Richmond Lattimore (Ann Arbor: University of Michigan Press, 1959), 24.

6. Walter Otto, *The Homeric Gods* (London: Thames and Judson, 1954), 97.

7. Paul Friedrich, *The Meaning of Aphrodite* (Chicago: University of Chicago Press, 1978), 89.

8. As quoted by Otto, *Homeric Gods,* 101.

9. Kenneth Clark, *The Nude: A Study in Ideal Form* (New York: Pantheon Books, 1956), 101.

10. Gadamer, *Truth and Method,* 434. Gadamer tells us that the German word *schön* connotes that which is not part of the necessary or purposeful as distinguished from technology or the useful.

11. James Hillman, *The Thought of the Heart* (Dallas: Spring Publications, 1981), 29.

12. "To Aphrodite," no. 5: 50.

13. As quoted by Hillman in *Heart,* 28.

14. Robert Sardello, the contemporary cultural psychologist, remarks that the

pornography of an imagination that denigrates physical appearance is reflected in the bare Aphrodite literalized in newstand pictures. See also Adolf Portmann's *Animal Forms and Patterns* (New York: Schocken Books, 1967) for an account of display as instinct in the animal world.

15. Clark, *The Nude,* 83.
16. Lingis, *Excesses,* 59–62.
17. Otto, *Homeric Gods,* 101.
18. Clark, *The Nude,* 102.
19. As quoted by Friedrich, *Meaning,* 77.
20. Carl Kerenyi, *Goddesses of Sun and Moon* (Dallas: Spring Publications, 1979), 41.
21. Carl Kerenyi, "Eidolon, Eikon, Agalme," in *Spring,* 1984 (Dallas: Spring Publications, 1984), 174–79.
22. "To Aphrodite," no. 6: 54.
23. Paris, *Meditations,* 23. Paris notes that it is a symptom of the pathology of our times that we transform gold into bars and hoard it underground.
24. Hillman, *Heart,* 28.
25. "To Aphrodite," no. 5: 47.
26. Rudolf Steiner tells of a legend in which Christ, when passing by a dead dog lying on the roadside, admired the beauty of its teeth.
27. As quoted by Paris, *Meditations,* 17.
28. Hillman, *Heart,* 25.

## CHAPTER 2. BEAUTY AS LIGHT

1. Heraclitus wrote, "You could not find the limits of soul, even though you travelled every road to do so." Fragment no. 42 as translated by Phillip Whellwright in *Heraclitus* (New York: Atheneum, 1964), 58.
2. Plato, *Phaedrus,* trans. R. Hackforth, in *The Collected Dialogues of Plato.*
3. As quoted by Giorgio de Santillana in "The Role of Art in the Scientific Renaissance," *Critical Problems in the History of Science,* ed. Marshal Clagett (Madison: University of Wisconsin Press, 1969), 64.
4. Marsilio Ficino, *Commentary on Plato's Symposium on Love,* trans. Sears Jayne (Dallas: Spring Publications, 1985), 47.
5. A. Hilary Armstrong, "The Divine Enhancement of Earthly Beauties," in *Beauty of the World,* Eranos Jahrbuch, 1984, ed. Rudolf Ritsema (Ascona, Switzerland: Eranos Foundation, 1985), 64.
6. Ibid., 51.
7. Ibid., 56.
8. Ibid., 59.
9. Plato, *Philebus,* trans. R. Hackforth, in *The Collected Dialogues of Plato.*
10. See E. R. Dodds, *Pagan and Christian in an Age of Anxiety* (New York: W. W. Norton and Company, 1965).
11. Porphyry, "On the Life of Plotinus and the Arrangement of his Work," in *Plotinus, The Enneads,* 1.
12. Armstrong, *Beauty,* 76.
13. Ibid., 51.
14. Ibid., 56.
15. Ibid., 77–78.

16. Heidegger, in his chapter "Plato's *Phaedrus:* Beauty and Truth in Felicitous Discordance" (in *The Will to Power as Art,* vol. 1 of *Nietzsche,* trans. David Krell [New York: Harper and Row] translates the phrase as, "The beautiful itself is given (to us men, here) by means of the most luminous mode of perception at our disposal, and we possess the beautiful as what most brightly glistens." Heidegger asserts that transla' tions that emphasize beauty in itself are misleading. "Plato does not mean that the beautiful itself, as an object, is 'perspicuous and lovely.' It is rather what is most luminus and what thereby draws us on and liberates us (196–97).

17. Hillman, *Heart,* 23.

18. Stanley Rosen, *Plato's Symposium* (New Haven: Yale University Press, 1968), 199–200.

19. Ernst Cassirer, *The Individual and the Cosmos in Renaissance Philosophy,* trans. Mario Domandi (New York: Harper and Row, 1964), 23.

20. As quoted in Cassirer, *The Individual,* 28.

21. Ibid., 53.

22. Ibid., 28.

23. Ibid., 32. In like mind, Yeats wrote, "I'm looking for the face I had before the world was made."

24. Erwin Panofsky, *Studies in Iconology* (New York: Oxford University Press, 1938), 137.

25. John Sallis, in *Being and Logos: The Way of Platonic Dialogue* (Pittsburgh: Duquesne University Press, 1970), distinguishes three kinds of movement in Socrates' sense of the soul—embodiment, procession, and ascendance to the divine banquet.

26. In this depiction of the soul, one can discern a prefiguration of Freud's tripartite characterization of the psyche as id, ego, and superego, just as in the Diotima's characterization of the progression toward beauty in the *Symposium,* one can discern a prefiguration of Freud's notion of sublimation.

27. The two-form nature of love is prefigured in Plato (*Sym. 180 d–e) and Plotinus* (*En.* 3.5.4).

28. Ficino, *Commentary,* 130.

29. Ibid., 118.

30. Ibid., 86.

31. Ibid., 86.

32. *The Letters of Marsilio Ficino* (London: Fellowship of the School of Economic Science, 1975), 86.

33. Gadamer, *Truth and Method,* 443.

34. James Hillman, *Re-Visioning,* xi.

35. Dante's description of achieving the "Beatific Vision" at the climax of *Paradiso* is similar. When he gazes into the "Light Eternal" (33, 124) and sees "Our likeness," (33, 131) he has "become very vision" in Plotinus's words.

36. William Blake, "Anguries of Innocence" 1.1.

37. Heidegger, *Nietzsche,* 192.

38. Hillman, *Heart.*

39. Sallis, *Being and Logos,* 149–50.

40. In his depiction of the "Beatific Vision," Dante wrote, "O Light Eternal, that alone abidest in / Thyself alone knowest Thyself, and known to / Thyself and knowing, lovest and smilest on Thyself!" (*Paradiso* 33, 124–26).

41. Gadamer, *Truth and Method,* 438.

42. Ibid., 441.

43. Ibid., 443.

44. Ibid., 442.

45. The medieval Christian world was one filled with references to divinity. In this sense the visible beauty of the earth was a matrix of signs pointing to the heavens. Through light, God was invested in all things. Visible beauty was an image of invisible beauty so that all things of the world took on a deeper significance. In the twelfth century, Suger, Abbot of St. Denis, made his monastery into a "House of God" in which jewelry and objects of art were stored. Suger describes his inventory as "a big golden chalice of 140 ounces of gold adorned with precious gems, viz., hyacinths and topazes, as a substitute for another one which had been lost as a pawn in the time of our predecessor . . . [and] . . . a porphyry vase, made admirable by the hand of the sculptor and polisher, after it had lain idly in a chest for many years, converting it from a flagon into the shape of an eagle." As quoted by Umberto Eco in *Art and Beauty in the Middle Ages* (New Haven: Yale University Press, 1986), 13, from Erwin Panofsky, *Abbot Suger on the Abbey Church of St. Denis and Its Art Treasures* (Princeton, 1946), 77, 79.

Suger tells of his pleasure in the physical ornamentation of the church.

Often we contemplate, out of sheer affection for the church our mother, these different ornaments both old and new; and when we behold how that wonderful cross of St. Eloy— together with the smaller ones—and that incomparable ornament commonly called "the crest" are placed upon the golden altar, then I say, sighing deeply in my heart: "Every precious stone was thy covering, the sardius, the topaz, and the jasper, the chrysolite, and the onyx, and the beryl, the sapphire, and the carbuncle, and the emerald. (As quoted by Eco, *Art and Beauty*, 6.)

These are the words of a man taken with love of the life inherent in things them-selves.

In like manner, the duc du Berry had a wide assortment of collectibles, which gives evidence of his sense of beauty in the things of the world. "The duc du Berry's collection included the horn of a unicorn, St. Joseph's engagement ring, coconuts, whale's teeth, and shells from the Seven Seas. It comprised around three thousand items. Seven hundred were paintings, but it also contained an embalmed elephant, an hydra, a basilisk, an egg which an Abbot had found inside another egg, and manna which had fallen during a famine" (Eco, *Art and Beauty*, 14).

For my purposes, the most important implication of the ontology of light is that it directs consciousness toward and honors body, earth, and the things of the world. This attitude emerges especially in Hugh of St. Victor. "Look upon the world and all that is in it: you will find much that is beautiful and desirable. . . . Gold . . . has its brilliance, the flesh its comeliness, clothes and ornaments their color" (as quoted by Eco, *Art and Beauty*, 10). St. Bernard saw the body as a sort of crystal, scattering rays of light. "When the brightness of beauty has replenished to overflowing the recesses of the heart, it is necessary that it should emerge into the open, just like the light hidden under a bushel: a light shining in the dark is not trying to conceal itself. The body is an image of the mind, which, like an effulgent light scattering forth its rays, is diffused through its members and sense, shining through in action, discourse, apearance movement—even in laughter, if it is completely sincere and tinged with gravity" (as quoted by Eco, *Art and Beauty*, 10).

St. Bonaventure took up the metaphysics of light. "Light is common by nature to all bodies celestial and terrestrial. . . . Light is the substantial form of bodies, by their greater or lesser participation in light, bodies, acquire *the truth and dignity of their being*" (as quoted by Eco, *Art and Beauty*, 50, italics mine).

For Albertus Magnus, beauty existed as a transcendent, objective quality, trans-

forming the multiple forms into a unity. He wrote, "The nature of the beautiful consists in general in a resplendence of form, whether in the daily-ordered parts of material objects or in men or in actions" (as quoted by Eco, *Art and Beauty*, 57).

46. Dionyius the Areopagite, *The Divine Names and the Mystical Theology*, trans. C. E. Rolt (New York: Macmillan, 1940), 91. This is one of the earliest uses of the word *archetype* cited by Jung. The idea of archetype is a cornerstone in Jungian and imaginal psychology, giving indication of the influence of the tradition of light on these two contemporary schools of depth psychology.

47. Ibid., 92.

48. Ficino, *Commentary*, 51–52.

49. Tom Moore, *The Planets Within* (Lewisburg, Pa.: Bucknell University Press, 1982) 91–92, paraphrasing from Ficino's *Opera Omnia*, 2 vols. (Basel, 1576; reprinted, Torino: Bottega d'Erasmo, 1959) 978.

50. In the thirteenth century, John Duns Scotus took great delight in multiplicity and the emphasis on the particularity of things. He thought that in a composite being, such as a human, there can be several *esse* corresponding to the different entities making up the composite. This emphasis on multiplicity is a forerunner to archetypal psychology, which emphasizes the many personalities in the psyche as opposed to a unitary self. See Hillman, *Re-Visioning*, 167–71.

Scotus also created a doctrine of *haeccitas* or "thisness." *Haeccitas* is a property of an object that confers concrete individuality. Whereas the Thomistic perspective focused on the catagory of a thing, for Scotus, the emphasis was on the uniqueness of each thing. Scotus's notion of *haeccitas* prefigures Jung's notion of individuation. For a discussion of Scotus, see Eco, *Art and Beauty*, 85–88.

51. Dionysius, *Divine Names*, 95–96.

52. Ficino, *Commentary*, 51–52.

53. Ficino, *Letters*, 84.

54. In the medieval and early Renaissance mind, color was the essence, not an attribute, of a substance. Therefore, the appearance of color was taken as indicating something essential and substantial about an object.

55. C. G. Jung, *Aion: Research into the Phenomenology of the Self*, collected works, Volume 9, part 2, trans. R. F. C. Hull (Princeton: Princeton University Press, 1959), 8–10.

56. Wheelwright, Fragment No. 2, p. 19.

57. Dionysius, *Divine Names*, 96.

58. Gadamer, 439.

59. Wheelwright, fragment no. 106, 90.

60. Gadamer, *Truth and Method*, 437, 439.

61. As quoted by Michael Allen in *The Platonism of Marsilio Ficino* (Berkeley: University of California Press, 1984), 191.

62. Even outside of the Neoplatonic tradition, appearance, perception, and being can be equated. Aristotle asserts, "What appears to all, this we call Being" (*Nicomachean Ethics* 1172 b 36). Likewise, George Berkeley declares, "*Essi es percipi*" in A *Treatise Concerning the Principles of Human Knowledge*, 1, 3).

63. Dionysius, *Divine Names*, 96.

64. Ibid., 6.

65. Ibid., 100.

66. Heidegger, *Nietzsche*, vol. 1, 97.

67. See Kerenyi, "Eidolon, Eikon, Agalma," for an explanation of the concealing aspect of image.

68. James Hillman, "Senex and Puer," in *Puer Papers*, Hillman et. al. (Dallas: Spring Publications, 1979), 12.

69. As quoted by Martin Heidegger in "What Are Poets For?" in *Poetry, Language, Thought,* 124.
70. As quoted by James Hillman in "Senex and Puer," 15.

# CHAPTER 3. APHRODITE REFUSED

1. St. Augustine, *The Confessions of St. Augustine,* trans. Ray Warner (New York: The New American Library, 1963), 215.
2. Ibid., 235.
3. Ibid.
4. Elaine Pagels, "The Politics of Paradise," *The New York Review of Books,* 12 May 1988; Dodds, *Anxiety,* 1–36; Hannah Arendt, *The Life of the Mind: Willing* (New York: Harcourt Brace Jovanovich, 1978), 67ff.
5. Pagels, "Politics," 28.
6. Arendt, *Willing,* 67.
7. Ibid., 74.
8. Ibid., 78.
9. Ibid., 71.
10. As quoted by Geoffrey Grigson, *The Goddess of Love* (New York: Stein and Day, 1977), 229.
11. As quoted by Paris, *Meditations, 38.*
12. *As quoted by Dodds, Anxiety, 32.*
13. As quoted by Grigson, *Goddess,* 141.
14. Arnobius of Sicca, *The Case Against the Pagans,* trans. George F. McCracken (Westminster, Md.: Newman Press, 1949), 213.
15. Clement of Alexandria, "The Exhortation to the Greeks," in *Clement of Alexandra,* trans. G. W. Butterworth (New York: G. P. Putnam's Sons, 1919), 55.
16. Ibid., 5.
17. Ibid., 33.
18. As quoted by Grigson, *Goddess,* 139.
19. Clement of Alexandria, "Exhortation," 75.
20. Ibid., 137.
21. Clement of Alexandria, *Christ the Educator,* trans. Simon Wood (New York: Fathers of the Church, 1954), 134.
22. Ibid., 146.
23. As quoted in John Ferguson, *Clement of Alexandria* (New York: Twayne Publishers), 194.
24. Clement of Alexandria, *Christ,* 190.
25. Ibid., 194.
26. Clement of Alexandria, "Exhortation," 133.
27. See J. Martin, *A History of the Iconoclast in Controversy* (New York, 1931); Paul Alexander, *The Patriarch Nicephorus of Constantinope: Ecclesiastical Policy and Image Worship in the Byzantine Empire* (Oxford, 1958); *Iconoclasm: Papers Given at the Ninth Spring Symposium of Byzantine Studies, University of Birmingham,* ed. Anthony Bryer and Judith Herrin (Birmingham, England, 1977); Jaroslav Pelikan, *Imago Dei: The Byzantine Apologia for Icons* (Princeton: Princeton University Press, 1987).
28. Martin Luther, "Treatise on Christian Liberty," trans. W. A. Lambert, in *Works of Martin Luther,* edited by the Board of Publication, United Lutheran Church in America (Philadelphia: Muhlenberg Press, 1943), 313.
29. Steven Ozment, "Luther and the Late Middle Ages: The Formation of Refor-

mation Thought," in *Transition and Revolution: Problems and Issues of European Renaissance and Reformation History,* ed. Robert M. Kingdom (Minneapolis: Burgess, 1974), 126.

30. As quoted by Ozment, "Reformation Thought," 126.

31. Ibid.

32. As quoted by Edward Dowden in *Puritan and Anglican,* (Freeport, N.Y.: Books for Libraries Press, 1901), 10.

33. Blake held the opposite view, that it was reason that was satanic and the imagination that was Christ-like. See *The Marriage of Heaven and Hell.*

34. Dodds, *Anxiety,* 24.

35. Clark, *The Nude,* 95.

36. J. H. Van den Berg, *The Changing Nature of Man: Introduction to a Historical Psychology* (New York: Dell Publishing Company, 1975), 230–31. See also Robert Romanyshyn, *Psychological Life, From Science to Metaphor* (Austin: University of Texas Press, 1982), 24–26.

37. Clark, *The Nude,* 103.

## CHAPTER FOUR. PROPORTION: BEAUTY AS MEASURE

1. As quoted in Eco, *Art and Beauty,* 28.

2. As quoted by Erwin Panofsky in "The History of the Theory of Human Proportions as a Reflection of the History of Styles" in *Meaning in the Visual Arts* (Chicago: University of Chicago Press, 1984), 68.

3. Ibid., 69.

4. W. K. C. Guthrie, *The Greek Philosophers* (New York: Harper Colophon Books, 1975), 36.

5. Ibid., 40.

6. Plato, *Philebus,* trans. R. Hackforth, in *The Collected Dialogues of Plato.*

7. Aristotle's notion of beauty follows Plato's emphasis on measure and proportion. "Now the most important kinds of the beautiful are order (*taxis*), symmetry (*summetra*) and definiteness (*horismon*) and the mathematical sciences exhibit properties of these in the highest degree: (*Metaphysics* 1078 a 30). "To be beautiful, a living creature and every whole made up of parts must not only present a certain order in its arrangement of parts, but also be of a certain definite magnitude. Beauty is a matter of size and order" (*Poetics* 1450 b 4). Whereas Plato saw the standards and measurements which are the criteria for what is beautiful as derivations of the divine ideal, Aristotle considered beauty as a property of art work or natural objects. Aristotle separated beauty from the divine, and in doing so, separated beauty from the good (*Metaphysics* 1978 a 30) and the useful (*Metaphysics* 1333a).

One can see here, at first in Plato and then in Aristotle, the beginnings of the diminishment of beauty as a psychological value in and of itself. As earthly beauty is considered separate from the divine and considered only in terms of measure, it becomes a spiritual attribute pointing to divine forms of perfection. Beauty as an abstraction, that is, measure, has a diminished psychological value because it refers away from the concrete to a "higher" conceptual order. This is a notion that limits beauty to symmetrical perfection and, as Plotinus points out, leaves out all of the nonsymmetrical forms that move the soul.

8. Plato, *Republic,* trans. Paul Shorey, in *The Collected Dialogues of Plato.*

9. As quoted from Monroe C. Beardsley in "Aesthetics, History of," in *The*

*Encyclopedia of Philosophy,* ed. Paul Edwards (New York: Macmillan Company, 1967), 23.

10. St. Augustine, "De Musica," in *Philosophies of Art and Beauty,* trans. Robert Russell, ed. Albert Hofstadter and Richard Kuhns (Chicago: University of Chicago Press, 1976), 194.

11. Ibid., 186–87.

12. Ibid., 191.

13. Ibid., 184–85.

14. St. Augustine, "De Ordine," trans. Robert P. Russell, in *Philosophies of Art and Beauty,* 181.

15. Ibid., 174.

16. St. Augustine, "De Musica," 186.

17. St. Augustine, "De Ordine," 180.

18. Ibid., 182.

19. Ibid., 183.

20. St. Augustine, "De Musica," 191.

21. Gadamer, *Truth and Method,* 440.

22. St. Augustine, "De Ordine," 181.

23. Eco, *Art and Beauty,* 30.

24. St. Augustine, "De Ordine," 178.

25. St. Augustine, "De Musica," 195.

26. As quoted in Guthrie, *Greek Philosophers,* 40.

27. St. Augustine, "De Musica," 200.

28. Arendt considers Augustine the "first philosopher of the Will" in *Willing.*

## CHAPTER 5. LINEAR PERSPECTIVE

1. See Jacob Burckhardt, "The Discovery of the World and of Man," part 4 of *The Civilization of the Renaissance in Italy* (New York: MacMillan, 1921).

2. See Burckhardt, *Civilization,* 328, regarding the beginnings of biography; and Nesca Robb, *The Neoplatonism of the Italian Renaissance* (New York: Octagon Books, 1968), 43, for a discussion of "personality" as the "final miracle of beauty in a glorious universe."

3. See Eco, *Art and Beauty,* 92–93.

4. Ernst Cassirer, *The Individual and the Cosmos in Renaissance Philosophy,* trans. Mario Domandi (New York: Harper and Row, 1964), 92.

5. Panofsky, "Human Proportions," 90–92.

6. As quoted by Eco, *Art and Beauty,* 67.

7. St. Thomas, *Summa Theologiae,* trans. Timothy McDermott (New York: McGraw-Hill, 1964), 73.

8. As quoted in Eco, *Art and Beauty,* 67, from William of Auvergne, *De Bono et Male.*

9. See "The Fathers of Optics," in Samual Edgerton, *The Renaissance Rediscovery of Linear Perspective* (New York: Basic Books, 1975), 60–78. Although the history of the metaphysics of light and optics extended from the ancient Greek philosophers through Arab and medieval Christian philosophers, in the thirteenth century there was renewed interest regarding what was happening in the eye of the perceiver from both a theological and a mathematical standpoint.

10. As quoted by Eco, *Art and Beauty,* 49, from *Hexaemeron.*

11. As quoted by Edgerton, *Linear Perspective,* 74.

12. As quoted from Alberti by Erwin Panofsky, *The Life and Art of Albrecht Dürer*

(Princeton: Princeton University Press, 1955), 247.

13. As quoted from Manetti by Giorgio de Santillana in "The Role of Art in the Scientific Renaissance," in *Critical Problems in the History of Science,* ed. Marshall Clagett (Madison: University of Wisconsin Press, 1969), 64.

14. In contrast, Raphael is known to have said that in matters of beauty, he trusted in a certain idea that came into his mind and of which he did not know whether or not it had artistic excellence. See Panofsky, *Dürer,* 274.

15. As quoted in Edgerton, *Linear Perspective,* 30.

16. Ibid., 86.

17. Ibid., 30.

18. Ibid., 92–93.

19. As quoted by Panofsky in *Dürer,* 275.

20. Ibid., 277.

21. Ibid.

22. Ibid., 281.

23. See de Santillana, "Role of Art."

24. Robert Romanyshyn, *Psychological Life,* 175. See also Robert Romanyshyn, *Technology as Symptom and Dream* (New York: Routledge, 1989) for an account of how linear perspective has shaped the modern identity through technological vision.

25. Thomas Kuhn, *The Structure of Scientific Revolutions* (Chicago: University of Chicago Press, 1970).

26. As quoted by de Santillana, *"Role of Art,"* 35.

27. Ibid., 54.

# CHAPTER 6. THE SUBJECTIVIZATION OF BEAUTY

1. Cassirer discusses the subject-object problem in the philosophy of the Renaissance in chapter 4 of *Individual and Cosmos.*

2. Heidegger, *Nietzsche,* 83.

3. Rodolphe Gasche, *Tain of the Mirror, Derrida and the Philosophy of Reflection* (Cambridge: Harvard University Press, 1986), 14.

4. Panofsky, "Human Proportions," 105.

5. As quoted by Armaud Maurer in *About Beauty: A Thomistic Interpretation* (Houston: Center for Thomistic Studies, 1983), 33.

6. Jerome Stolnitz, "On the Origins of 'Aesthetic Disinterestedness'," in *Aesthetics, A Critical Anthology,* ed. George Dickie and R. J. Sclafani (New York: St. Martin's Press, 1977).

7. From Shaftesbury's *Characteristics* 1, 274, as quoted in Stolnitz in "Origins," 610.

8. Stolnitz, "Origins," 610.

9. Ibid.

10. Ibid., 621.

11. Ibid.

12. Francis Hutcheson, "An Initial Theory of Taste," from *An Inquiry into the Original of our Ideas of Beauty and Virtue* (1725), in *Aesthetics: A Critical Anthology,* 574.

13. Ibid., 577.

14. Ibid., 572.

15. Ibid., 587.

16. Ibid., 570.

17. Ibid., 575.

18. Stolnitz, "Origins," 622.

19. Ibid., 621.

20. Ibid., 622.

21. As quoted by Jerome Stolnitz in "Beauty: Some stages in the History of an Idea," *Journal of the History of Ideas* 22, no. 2 (1961): 185–204.

22. As quoted by Jerome Stolnitz in "Beauty," in *The Encyclopedia of Philosophy*, ed. Paul Edwards (New York: Macmillan, 1967), 265.

23. Edmund Burke, *A Philosophical Enquiry into the Origin of our Ideas of the Sublime and the Beautiful* (1757) (Notre Dame: University of Notre Dame Press, 1978), 66.

24. Ibid., 106.

25. Ibid., 115.

26. Ibid., 116.

27. Ibid., 112.

28. From Alison's *Essays in the Nature and Principles of Taste*, as quoted by Stolnitz, in "Origins," 616.

29. Ibid.

30. Stolnitz, "Origins," 575.

31. David Hume, "Of the Standard of Taste" (1657), in *Aesthetics: A Critical Anthology*, 594.

32. Ibid., 601.

33. Immanuel Kant, *The Critique of Judgement*, trans. James Meredith (Oxford: Clarendon Press, 1928), 41.

34. Ibid., 41–42.

35. Ibid.

36. Gadamer, *Truth and Method*, 38.

37. Ibid., 38–39.

38. Kant, *Critique*, 58.

39. Gadamer, *Truth and Method*, 40.

40. Kant, *Critique*, 58.

41. Ibid., 151.

42. Ibid., 153.

43. Kant, *Critique*, 42.

44. Ibid., 49.

45. Ibid., 43.

46. Ibid., 47.

47. Ibid., 43.

48. Robert Zimmerman, "Kant: The Aesthetic Judgement," *Journal of Aesthetics and Art Criticism* 21, no. 3 (Spring 1963): 334.

49. Ibid., 340.

50. Heidegger, *Nietzsche*, 112.

51. Ibid., 108.

52. Ibid., 109.

53. Kant, *Critique*, 48.

54. Ibid., 49.

55. Ibid., 149.

56. Ibid., 54.

57. Ibid., 61–62.

58. Ibid., 75–76.

59. Ibid., 76.

60. Ibid.

61. Gadamer, *Truth and Method*, 45.
62. Kant, *Critique*, 223–24.
63. Gadamer, *Truth and Method*, 76.


# CHAPTER 7. IMAGE IN DEPTH PSYCHOLOGY

1. Arendt, *Human Condition*, 275.
2. Michael Polanyi has given insight into the aesthetic ground that he sees underlying scientific understanding in his book *Personal Knowledge, Towards A Post-Critical Philosophy* (Chicago: The University of Chicago Press, 1958). Polanyi writes, "We cannot truly account for our acceptance of such theories [modern physics] without endorsing our acknowledgement of beauty that exhilarates and a profundity that entrances us" (15). In Polanyi's account of the "tacit" dimension in scientific knowledge, he emphasizes passion for "intellectual beauty" as a guide to that which the scientist assigns value. "I want to show that this appreciation depends ultimately on a sense which can never be dispassionately defined, any more than we can dispassionately define the beauty of a work of art or the excellence of a noble action" (135). In other words, it is the scientist's sense of the beauty of a theory that evokes his passion thus revealing to him his sense of truth.
3. Alan Megill, *Prophets of Extremity: Nietzsche, Heidegger, Foucault, Derrida* (Berkeley: University of California Press, 1985), 36.
4. Ibid., 37.
5. Friederich Nietzsche, *The Birth of Tragedy and the Genealogy of Morals*, trans. Francis Golfing (Garden City, N.Y.: Doubleday, 1956), 9.
6. Ibid., 29.
7. Friederich Nietzsche, "On Truth and Falsity in an Extra-Moral Sense," in *Nietzsche, Early Greek Philosophy and Other Essays*, trans. M. A. Mügge, vol. 2 of *The Complete Works of Friederich Nietzsche*, ed. Oscar Levy, (New York: Russell and Russell, 1964), 179. Following Megill, I have used his altered translation substituting the word *concept* for Mügge's *idea* when Nietzsche uses the word *Begriff*. *Idea* is inappropriate because its root is *eidos*, meaning "image," and in using *Begriff*, Nietzsche intends the opposite of image.
8. Ibid., 184.
9. Ibid., 183.
10. Ibid., 178.
11. Ibid., 180.
12. Ibid., 184.
13. Ibid., 181.
14. Ibid., 184.
15. Ibid., 190.
16. Ibid.
17. As quoted by Heidegger in *Nietzsche*, 112.
18. William Blake, *Jerusalem* 69.25.
19. Ibid., 98.30–31.
20. William Blake, "A Vision of the Last Judgement" 69.
21. William Blake, [The Laocoön] as published in *The Poetry and Prose of William Blake*, ed. David Erdman (Garden City, N.Y.: Doubleday, 1970) 271.
22. As quoted by Northrup Frye in *Fearful Symmetry* (Princeton: Princeton University Press, 1947), 30, from Blake's margin notes to Berkeley as published in vol. 3 of *The Writings of William Blake*, ed. Geoffrey Keynes (London, 1925), 356. See also

Kathleen Raine, "William Blake: The Beautiful and the Holy," *Dragonflies: Studies in Imaginal Psychology* vol. II, no. 2, (Summer 1980): 19–36, for a study of imagination and beauty in Blake.

23. Ibid., 25.

24. Ibid., 259.

25. Sigmund Freud, *The Interpretation of Dreams*, trans. James Strachey (New York: Avon Books, 1965), 82.

26. Ibid.

27. Ibid., 581.

28. Ibid., 224.

29. Ibid., 608.

30. Sigmund Freud, *New Introductory Lectures on Psychoanalysis*, trans. James Strachey (New York: W. W. Norton and Co., 1965), 16.

31. Sigmund Freud, *A General Introduction to Psychoanalysis* (New York: Washington Square Press, 1952), 189.

32. Sigmund Freud, *An Outline of Psycho-Analysis*, trans. James Strachey (New York: W. W. Norton and Co., 1969), 22.

33. Freud, *New Introductory Lectures*, 10.

34. Freud, *Interpretation*, 44, 177, 603, and *New Introductory Lectures*, 11.

35. Freud, *Interpretation*, 128, 132.

36. Freud, *A General Introduction*, 179.

37. See Patricia Berry-Hillman's *Jung's Early Psychiatric Writing: The Emergence of a Psychopoetics* (Ph.D. diss., University of Dallas, 1984) for a history and analysis of Jung's ambivalent attitude toward aesthetics in the formative stages of his career.

38. C. G. Jung, *Memories, Dreams, Reflections*, recorded and edited by Aniela Jaffe, trans. Richard and Clara Winston (New York: Vintage Books, 1961), 16.

39. Ibid., 187.

40. C. G. Jung, *Psychological Types*, Collected Works, volume 6, trans. R. F. C. Hull, (Princeton: Princeton University Press), 140.

41. Ibid., 142.

42. C. G. Jung, *The Structure and Dynamics of the Psyche*, collected works, volume 8, trans. R. F. C. Hull (Princeton, N.J.: Princeton University Press, 1960), 263.

43. C. G. Jung, *The Practice of Psychotherapy*, collected works, volume 16, trans. R. F. C. Hull (Princeton: Princeton University Press, 1966), 151.

44. Jung, *Structure*, 263.

45. Jung, *Practice*, 151.

46. Patricia Berry, "An Approach to the Dream," in *Spring, 1974* (New York: Spring Publications, 1974), 58–79.

47. C. G. Jung, *Two Essays on Analytical Psychology*, collected works, volume 7, trans. R. F. C. Hall (Princeton: Princeton University Press, 1966), 177.

48. Jung, *Structure*, 248.

49. Ibid., 287.

50. ibid., 277.

51. Jung, *Types*, 540.

52. Ibid., 555.

53. See James Hillman's *Egalitarian Typologies Versus the Perception of the Unique* (Dallas: Spring Publications, 1980) for a full discussion of typological versus aesthetic vision. Hillman cites research in which G. W. Allport and H. S. Odbert ("Trait-Names: A Psycho-lexical Study," *Psychological Monographs, Psychological Review* 47,1, no. 211 [1936]: 8) compile 17,953 personality trait names.

54. Jung, *Two Essays*, 72.

55. Ibid., 221.

56. Ibid.

57. Jung's notion of compensation in dream interpretation was formulated as early as 1916 in "General Aspects of Dream Psychology" (CW 8). *Psychological Types* (CW 8) was written during the period of 1913–18. Energic formulations were conceived in 1912 in "On Psychic Energy" (CW 8) and in 1916 in "The Transcendent Function" (CW 8). Initial formulations of the self as midpoint of the psyche appeared in 1916/1928 in "The Relation Between the Ego and the Unconscious" (CW 7).

58. *Dream Analysis, Notes of the Seminar Given in 1928–1930 by C. G. Jung,* ed. William McGuire (Princeton: Princeton University Press, 1984), 204.

59. C. G. Jung, *Civilization in Transition* collected works, volume 10, trans., R. F. C. Hull (Princeton: Princeton University Press, 1958), 49.

60. Jung, *Practice,* 149.

61. Jung, *Structure,* 284.

62. Ibid., 201.

63. Ibid., 204.

64. Ibid., 86.

65. Ibid., 90.

66. Jung, *Types,* 476.

67. Jung, *Structure,* 90.

68. Ibid., 353.

69. Ibid., 384.

70. C. G. Jung, *Psychology and Religion,* collected works, volume 11, trans. R. F. C. Hull (Princeton: Princeton University Press, 1958), 480.

71. Ibid., 544.

72. Cited in "C. G. Jung on the Psychological," excerpted and arranged by Barbara Fisher Gilland Randolph Severson, *Spring, 1979,* 206.

73. Jung, *Alchemical Studies,* 50.

74. C. G. Jung, *Mysterium Coniunctionis,* collected works, volume 14, trans. R. F. C. Hull (Princeton: Princeton University Press, 1963), 180.

75. Jung, *Types,* 453.

76. Ibid., 52.

77. Ibid., 57.

78. Jung, *Two Essays,* 174.

79. Jung, *Types,* 44.


# CHAPTER 8. BEAUTY AND PSYCHOTHERAPY

1. Hannah Arendt, *The Human Condition* (Chicago: University of Chicago Press, 1958), 26.

2. Ibid., 27.

3. Ibid.

4. Ibid., 15.

5. Ibid., 47.

6. Ibid., 207–8.

7. As quoted by Erwin Panofsky, *Studies in Iconology: Humanistic Themes in the Art of the Renaissance* (New York: Oxford University Press, 1939), 140.

8. As quoted by Panofsky, *Studies,* 140.

9. Marsilio Ficino, vol. 1 of *The Letters of Marsilio Ficino* (London: Fellowship of the School of Economic Science, 1975), 81.

10. Arendt, *Human Condition,* 303.

11. Bruce Wilshire, *Role Playing and Identity: The Limits of Theatre as Metaphor* (Bloomington: Indiana University Press, 1982), 31.

12. Maurice Merleau-Ponty, *The Phenomenology of Perception* (New Jersey: Humanities Press, 1962), 184.

13. Ibid., 196.

14. Ibid., 182–83.

15. Heidegger, "Poetically," 226.

16. Gadamer, *Truth and Method,* 407.

17. Arendt, *Human Condition,* 192.

18. Gadamer, *Truth and Method,* 111.

19. Merleau-Ponty, *Phenomenology,* 68.

20. William Goodheart, "Theory of Analytic Interaction," *The San Francisco Jung Institute Library Journal* vol. 1, no. 4 (Summer 1980): 20.

21. William Goodheart, "Successful and Unsuccessful Interventions in Jungian Analysis: The Construction and Destruction of the Spellbinding Circle," in *Transference/Countertransference,* ed. Nathan Schwartz-Salant and Murray Stein (Wilmette, Illinois: Chiron Publications, 1984).

22. Sally Parks, "Experiments in Approaching A New Way of Listening," *Journal of Analytical Psychology* 32 (1987): 93–115.

23. See *Narcissism and Character Transformation* (Toronto: Inner City Books, 1982), and especially "Archetypal Factors Underlying Sexual Acting-out in the Transference/Countertransference Process," *Chiron: A Review of Jungian Analysis* vol. 1., (1984): 1–30, and "On the Subtle-Body Concept in Clinical Practice," in *The Body in Analysis,* ed. Nathan Schwartz-Salant and Murray Stein (Wilmette, Illinois: Chiron Publications, 1986).

24. Schwartz-Salant, "Subtle-Body," 19.

25. Ibid.

26. Ibid., 30.

27. Ibid., 33.

28. Ibid., 34.

29. Ibid.

30. Ibid.

31. Ibid., 38.

32. Ibid.

33. Ibid., 41.

34. Ibid., 43.

35. Ibid., 49.

36. Ibid., 50.

37. As quoted by Wilshire, *Role Playing,* 33.

# CHAPTER 9. TOWARD A PSYCHOLOGY OF APPEARANCE

1. Gaston Bachelard, *The Poetics of Reverie,* trans. Danial Russell (Boston: Beacon Press, 1969), 185.

2. Hillman, *Heart,* 34.

3. *Theaetetus* 155:d, trans. F. M. Cornford, in *The Collected Dialogue of Plato.*

4. Jung, *Practise,* 189.

5. Onians, *Origins,* 74–75.

6. James Joyce, *Finnegan's Wake* (New York: Viking, 1939), 378ff.

7. David Miller, *Christs* (New York: Seabury Press, 1981), 76.

8. Hillman, *Heart,* 34.

9. Gadamer, *Truth and Method,* 81.

10. Ibid., 130.

11. What I have been referring to as "beauty" is similar to what Robert Pirsig calls "Quality," the universal principle that contains the dualities of subject and object, art and science, in his novel, *Zen and the Art of Motorcycle Maintenance.*

12. James Hillman, "Image Sense," in *Spring, 1979* (Dallas: Spring Publications), 142.

13. Jung, *Structure,* 191.

14. Hillman, *Heart,* 29.

15. As quoted by Robert Avens, *The New Gnosis* (Dallas: Spring, 1984), 25.

16. Hillman, *Heart,* 25.

# BIBLIOGRAPHY

Adkins, Arthur. *Merit and Responsibility, A Study in Greek Values.* Oxford: Claren-don Press, 1960.

Allen, Michael. *The Platonism of Marsilio Ficino.* Berkeley: University of California Press, 1984.

Aquinas, Saint Thomas. *The Metaphysics of St. Thomas.* Translated by James Ander-son. Chicago: Henry Regnery Co., 1953.

————. *Summa Theologia.* Translated by Timothy McDermott. London: Blackfriars, 1961.

Arendt, Hannah. *The Human Condition.* Chicago: University of Chicago Press, 1958.

————. *The Life of the Mind.* Vol. 1, *Thinking.* New York: Harcourt Brace Jovanovich, 1978.

Aristotle. *Aristotle's On The Soul.* Translated by Hippocrates G. Apostle. Grinnel, Iowa: Peripatetic Press, 1981.

Armstrong, A. Hilary. "Beauty and the Discovery of Divinity in the Thought of Plotinus." In *Plotinian and Christian Studies.* London: Varorum, 1979.

————. "The Divine Enhancement of Earthly Beauties: The Hellenic and Platonic Tradition." In *Beauty of the World, Eranos Jaliubuch, 1984,* edited by Rudolf Ritsema. Ascona, Switzerland: Eranos, 1985.

Arnobius of Sicca. *The Case Against the Pagans.* Translated by George E. McCracken. Westminster, Maryland: Newman Press, 1949.

Augustine, Saint. *The Confessions of St. Augustine.* Translated by Rex Warner, New York: Mentor-Omega, 1963.

————. *De Musica.* Translated by W. F. Jackson Knight. In *Philosophies of Art and Beauty,* edited by Albert Hofstadter and Richard Kuhns. Chicago: University of Chicago Press, 1964.

————. *De Ordine.* Translated by Robert P. Russell. In *Philosophies of Art and Beauty,* edited by Albert Hofstadter and Richard Kuhns. Chicago: University of Chicago Press, 1964.

————. *"The Greatness of the Soul" and "The Teacher."* Translated by Joseph M. Colleran. Westminster, Md.: Newman Press, 1964.

Avens, Robert. *The New Gnosis.* Dallas: Spring Publications, 1984.

Bachelard, Gaston. *The Poetics of Reverie.* Translated by Daniel Russell. Boston: Beacon Press, 1969.

Beardsley, Monroe. "Aesthetics, History of." In *The Encyclopedia of Philosophy,* edited by Paul Edwards. New York: Macmillan, 1967.

Berry, Patricia. "An Approach to the Dream." In *Spring,* 1974. New York: Spring Publishing Company, 1974.

Berry-Hillman, Patricia. *Jung's Early Psychiatric Writing: The Emergence of a Psycho-poetics.* Ph.D. diss., University of Dallas, 1984.

Bettoni, Efram. *Duns Scotus: The Basic Principles of His Philosophy.* Translated and edited by Bernardine Bonansea. Washington D.C.: Catholic University of America Press, 1961.

Blake, William. *The Poetry and Prose of William Blake.* Edited by David Erdman, and commentary by Harold Bloom. Garden City, N.Y.: Doubleday, 1965.

Brehier, Emile. *The Philosophy of Plotinus.* Translated by Joseph Thomas. Chicago: University of Chicago Press, 1958.

Burch, Robert. "Kant's Theory of Beauty as Ideal Art." In *Aesthetics, A Critical Anthology,* edited by George Dickie and R. J. Sclafani. New York: St. Martin's Press, 1977.

Burckhardt, Jacob. *The Civilization of the Renaissance in Italy.* Translated by S. G. C. Middlemore. London: George Allen and Unwin, 1921.

Burke, Edmund. *A Philosophical Enquiry into the Origin of our Ideas of the Sublime and Beautiful.* Notre Dame: University of Notre Dame Press, 1968.

Candea, Virgil. "Iconoclasm." In *The Encyclopedia of Religion,* edited by Mircea Eliade. New York: Macmillan, 1986.

Casey, Edward. "Toward An Archetypal Imagination." In *Spring, 1974.* Dallas: Spring Publications, 1974.

Cassirer, Ernst. *The Individual and the Cosmos in Renaissance Philosophy.* Translated by Mario Domandi. New York: Harper and Row, 1964.

Clark, Kenneth. *The Nude: A Study in Ideal Form.* New York: Pantheon Books, 1956.

Clement of Alexandria. *Christ the Educator.* Trans. Simon Wood. New York: Fathers of the Church, 1954.

————. "The Exhortation to the Greeks." In *Clement of Alexandria,* translated by G. W. Butterworth. New York: G. P. Putnam and Sons, 1919.

Dante. *The Divine Comedy of Dante Alighieri: Paradiso.* Translated by John D. Sinclair. New York: Oxford University Press, 1939.

Danto, Arthur. *Nietzsche as Philosopher.* New York: Macmillan, 1965.

de Santillana, Giorgio. "The Role of Art in the Scientific Renaissance." In *Critical Problems in the History of Science,* edited by Marshal Clagett. Madison: University of Wisconsin Press, 1969.

Dickie, George, and R. J. Sclanfani, eds. *Aesthetics: A Critical Anthology.* New York: St. Martin's Press, 1977.

Dionysius the Areopagite. *"The Divine Names" and "The Mystical Theology."* Translated by C. E. Rolt. New York: Macmillan, 1940.

Dodds, E. R. *Pagan and Christian in an Age of Anxiety.* New York: W. W. Norton and Co., 1965.

Dover, K. J. *Greek Popular Morality in the Time of Plato and Aristotle.* Berkeley: University of California Press, 1974

Dowden, Edward. *Puritan and Anglican.* Freeport, N.Y.: Books for Libraries Press, 1901.

Downing, Christine. *The Goddess: Mythological Images of the Feminine.* New York: Crossroads, 1981.

Eco, Umberto. *Art and Beauty in the Middle Ages.* Translated by Hugh Bredin. New Haven: Yale University Press, 1986.

Edgerton, Samual. *The Renaissance Rediscovery of Linear Perspective.* New York: Harper and Row, 1975.

Farnell, Richard. *The Cults of the Greek States.* Chicago: Aegean Press, 1971.

Ferguson, John. *Clement of Alexandria.* New York: Twayne Publishers, 1936.

Ficino, Marsilio. *Commentary on Plato's Symposium on Love.* Translated by Sears Jayne. Dallas: Spring Publications, 1985.

————. Vol. 1 of *The Letters of Marsilio Ficino.* London: Fellowship of the School of Economic Science, 1975.

Freud, Sigmund. *A General Introduction to Psychoanalysis.* Translated by Joan Rivere. New York: Washington Square Press, 1952.

————. *The Interpretation of Dreams.* Translated by James Strachey. New York: Avon Books, 1965.

————. *An Outline of Psychoanalysis.* Translated by James Strachey. New York: W. W. Norton and Co., 1969.

————. *New Introductory Lectures on Psychoanalysis.* Translated by James Strachey. New York: W. W. Norton and Co., 1965.

Friedländer, Paul. *Plato: The Dialogues.* Translated by Hans Meyerhoff. Princeton: Princeton University Press, 1959.

Friedrich, Paul. *The Meaning of Aphrodite.* Chicago: University of Chicago Press, 1978.

Frye, Northrup. *Fearful Symmetry.* Princeton: Princeton University Press, 1947.

Gadamer, Hans-Georg. *Truth and Method.* New York: Crossroad, 1982.

Gasché, Rodolphe. *The Tain of the Mirror: Derrida and the Philosophy of Reflection.* Cambridge: Harvard University Press, 1968.

Goodheart, William. "Theory of Analytic Interaction," *The San Francisco Jung Institute Library Journal* 1, no. 4 (Summer 1980).

————. "Successful and Unsuccessful Interventions in Jungian Analysis: The Construction and Destruction of the Spellbinding Circle." In *Transference/Countertransference,* edited by Nathan Schwartz-Salant and Murray Stein. Wilmette, Illinois: Chiron Publications, 1984.

Graeser, Andrea. *Plotinus and the Stoics: A Preliminary Study.* Leiden, Holland: E. J. Brill, 1972.

Grigson, Geoffrey. *The Goddess of Love.* New York: Stein and Day, 1977.

Gruber, G. M. A. "Plato's Theory of Beauty." *The Monist* 37, no. 2 (1927).

Guthrie, W. K. C. *The Greek Philosophers from Thales to Aristotle.* New York: Harper and Row, 1975.

Hamilton, Edith, and Huntington Cairnes, eds. *Plato: Collected Dialogues.* Princeton: Princeton University Press, 1961.

Heidegger, Martin. *The Will to Power as Art.* Vol. 1 of *Nietzsche,* translated by David Krell. San Francisco: Harper and Row, 1971.

————. *On the Way to Language.* Translated by Peter Hertz. New York: Harper and Row, 1971.

————. *Poetry, Language, Thought.* Translated by Albert Hofstadter. New York: Harper and Row, 1971.

*Hesiod.* Translated by Richard Lattimore. Ann Arbor: University of Michigan Press. 1959.

Hillman, James. *Re-Visioning Psychology.* New York: Harper and Row, 1975.

————. "An Inquiry into Image." In *Spring 77.* Dallas: Spring Publications, 1977.

———. "Psychotherapy's Inferiority Complex." In *Eranos Jahrbuch 46–1977.* pp. 121–74. Frankfurt a/M: Insel Verlag, 1981.

———. "Further Notes on Image." In *Spring 78.* Dallas: Spring Publications, 1978.

———. "Image-Sense." In *Spring 79.* Dallas: Spring Publications, 1979.

———. *The Dream and the Underworld.* New York: Harper and Row, 1979.

———. *The Thought of the Heart.* Dallas: Spring Publications, 1981.

———. "Natural Beauty Without Nature." In *Spring 85.* Dallas: Spring Publications, 1985.

———. "Notes on White Supremacy." In *Spring, 1986.* Dallas: Spring Publications, 1986.

Hillman, James, Henry A. Murray, Tom Moore, James Baird, Thomas Cowan, Randolph Severson. *Puer Papers.* Dallas: Spring Publications, 1979.

Hofstdter, Albert, and Richard Kuhns, eds. *Philosophies of Art and Beauty.* Chicago: University of Chicago Press, 1976.

Homer. *The Homeric Hymns.* Translated by Thelma Sargent. New York: W. W. Norton and Co., 1973.

———. The Odyssey of Homer. Translated by Richard Lattimore. New York: Harper and Row, 1967.

Hughes, Merritt, ed. John Milton: Complet Poems and Major Prose. Milton, John. *John Milton: Complete Poems and Major Prose.* Edited by Merritt Hughes. Indianapolis: Bobbs-Merrill Educational Publishing, 1957.

Hume, David. "Of the Standard of Taste." In *Aesthetics, A Critical Anthology,* edited by George Dickie and R. J. Sclafani. New York: St. Martin's Press, 1977.

Hutcheson, Francis. "An Initial Theory of Taste." From *An Inquiry into the Original of our Ideas of Beauty and Virtue* (1725). In *Aesthetics: A Critical Anthology,* edited by George Dickie and R. J. Sclafani. New York: St. Martin's Press, 1977.

Joyce, James. *Finnegan's Wake.* New York: Viking, 1939.

Jung, C. G. *Civilization in Transition.* Princeton: Princeton University Press, 1958.

———. *Psychology and Religion: West and East.* Translated by R. F. C. Hull. Princeton: Princeton University Press, 1958.

———. *Aion: Researches into the Phenomenology of the Self.* Translated by R. F. C. Hull. Princeton: Princeton University Press, 1959.

———. *The Structure and Dynamics of the Psyche.* Translated by R. F. C. Hull. Princeton: Princeton University Press, 1960.

———. *Memories, Dreams, Reflections.* Recorded and edited by Aniela Jaffe, and translated by Richard and Clara Winston. New York: Vintage Books, 1965.

———. *Two Essays on Analytical Psychology.* Translated by R. F. C. Hull. Princeton: Princeton University Press, 1966.

———. *The Practice of Psychotherapy.* Translated by R. F. C. Hull. Princeton: Princeton University Press, 1966.

———. *Alchemical Studies.* Translated by R. F. C. Hull. Princeton: Princeton University Press, 1967.

———. *Mysterium Coniunctionis.* Translated by R. F. C. Hull. Princeton: Princeton University Press, 1970.

———. *Psychological Types.* Translated by R. F. C. Hull. Princeton: Princeton University Press, 1971.

Kant, Immanuel. *The Critique of Judgement*. Translated by James Meredith. Oxford: Clarendon Press, 1928.

Kerenyi, Karl. *Goddesses of Sun and Moon*. Irving, Tex.: Spring Publications, 1979.

———. *The Gods of the Greeks*. London: Thames and Hudson, 1979.

———. "Eidolon, Eikon, Agalma." *Spring, 1984*. Dallas: Spring Publications, 1984.

Kirk, G. S., and J. E. Raven. *The Presocratic Philosophers*. Cambridge: Cambridge University Press, 1966.

Kovach, Francis. *Philosophy of Beauty*. Norman: University of Oklahoma Press, 1974.

Kristeller, Paul. *The Philosophy of Marsilio Ficino*. Translated by Virginia Conant. Gloucester, Mass.: Peter Smith, 1964.

Kuhn, Thomas. *The Structure of Scientific Revolutions*. (Chicago: University of Chicago Press, 1970.

Lingis, Alphonso. *Excesses: Eros and Culture*. Albany: State University of New York Press, 1983.

Lopez-Pedraza, Rafael. "Moon Madness—Titanic Love, A Meeting of Pathology and Poetry." In *Images of the Untouched*, edited by Joanne Stroud and Gail Thomas. Dallas: Spring Publications, 1982.

Luther, Martin. "Treatise on Christian Liberty." In *Works of Martin Luther*. edited by Board of Publication, United Lutheran Church in America. Philadelphia: Muhlenberg Press, 1943.

MacKenna, Stephen, trans. *Plotinus: The Enneads*. London: Faber and Faber, 1956.

Maurer, Armand. *About Beauty: A Thomistic Interpretation*. Houston: Center for Thomistic Studies, 1983.

McCloskey, Mary. *Kant's Aesthetic*. Albany: State University of New York Press, 1987.

McGuire, William, ed. *Dream Analysis: Notes of the Seminar Given in 1928–1930 by C. G. Jung*. Princeton: Princeton University Press, 1984.

McKeon, Richard, ed. *Introduction to Aristotle*. Chicago: University of Chicago Press, 1973.

Megill, Alan. *Prophets of Extremity: Nietzsche, Heidegger, Foucalt, Derrida*. Berkeley: University of California Press, 1985.

Merleau-Ponty, Maurice. *Phenomenology of Perception*. New Jersey: Humanities Press, 1962.

———. *The Visible and the Invisible*. Evanston: Northwestern University Press, 1968.

Micklem, Neil. "The Intolerable Image, The Mythic Background of Psychosis." In *Spring 79*. Dallas: Spring Publications, 1979.

Miller, David. *Gods and Games*. New York: Harper and Row, 1973.

———. *Christs*. New York: Seabury Press, 1981.

Moore, Tom. *The Planets Within*. Lewisburg: Bucknell University Press, 1982.

Mothersill, Mary. *Beauty Restored*. Oxford: Clarendon Press, 1984.

Neumann, Erich. *Amor and Psyche*. Translated by Ralph Mannheim. Princeton: Princeton University Press, 1971.

Nietzsche, Friedrich. *"The Birth of Tragedy" and "The Genealogy of Morals."* Translated by Francis Golfing. Garden City, N.Y.: Doubleday, 1956.

———. "On Truth and Falsity in an Extra-Moral Sense." In *Nietzsche, Early Greek Philosophy and Other Essays*, translated by M. A. Mügge. Vol. 2 of *The Complete*

*Works of Friedrich Nietzsche,* edited by Oscar Levy. New York: Russell and Russell, 1964.

Onians, R. B. *The Origins of European Thought.* Cambridge: Cambridge University Press, 1954.

Otto, Walter. *The Homeric Gods.* London: Thames and Hudson, 1979.

Ozment, Steven. "Luther and the Late Middle Ages: The Formation of Reformation and Thought." In *Transition and Revolution: Problems and Issues of European Renaissance and Reformation History,* edited by Robert M. Kingdom. Minneapolis: Burgess, 1974.

Pagels, Elaine, "The Politics of Paradise," *The New York Times Review of Books,* 12 May 1988.

Panofsky, Erwin. *Studies in Iconology: Humanistic Themes in the Art of the Ranaissance.* New York: Oxford University Press, 1939.

———. *The Life and Art of Albrecht Dürer.* Princeton: Princeton University Press, 1955.

———. *Renaissance and Renascences.* New York: Harper and Row, 1972.

———. "The History of the Theory of Human Proportions as a Reflection of the History of Styles." In *Meaning in the Visual Arts.* Chicago: University of Chicago Press, 1982.

Paris, Ginette. *Pagan Meditations.* Dallas: Spring Publications, 1986.

Parks, Sally. "Experiments in Approaching A New Way Listening." *Journal of Analytical Psychology* 32 (1987): 93–115.

Pelikan, Jaroslav. *Imago Dei: The Byzantine Apologia for Icons.* Princeton: Princeton University Press, 1987.

Petrarca, Francesco. "The Ascent of Mont Ventoux." In *The Renaissance Philosophy of Man,* edited by Ernst Cassirer, Paul Kristeller, and John Randall, Jr. Chicago: University of Chicago Press, 1948.

Phelan, G. B. "The Concept of Beauty in St. Thomas Aquinas." In *Selected Papers,* edited by Arthur Kirn. Toronto: Pontifical Institute of Medieval Studies, 1967.

Pirsig, Robert M. *Zen and the Art of Motorcycle Maintenance.* New York: Bantam, 1974.

Pico della Mirandola, Giovanni. *On the Dignity of Man, On Being and the One, Heptaplus.* Edited by P. J. W. Miller. Indianapolis: Bobbs Merill, 1965.

Polanyi, Michael. *Personal Knowledge.* Chicago: University of Chicago Press, 1958.

Porphyry. "On the Life of Plotinus and the Arrangement of his Work." In *Plotinus, the Enneads,* translated by Stephen MacKenna. London: Faber and Faber, 1956.

Portmann, Adolf. *Animal Forms and Patterns.* New York: Schocken Books, 1967.

Raine, Kathleen. "The Use of the Beautiful." In *Defending Ancient Springs.* West Stockbridge, Mass.: Lindisfarne Press, 1967.

———. "William Blake: The Beautiful and the Holy." *Dragonflies: Studies in Imaginal Psychology* vol. 2, no. 2, (Summer 1980): 19–36.

Rist, John M. *Eros and Psyche: Studies in Plato, Plotinus and Origen.* Toronto: University of Toronto Press, 1964.

Robb, Nesca. *Neoplatonism of the Italian Renaissance.* New York: Octagon Books, 1968.

Rodgers, Priscilla. "The Healing Evocation of Beauty." In *Pratt Institute Creative Arts Therapy Review* 8 (1987).

Romanyshyn, Robert. *Psychological Life: From Science to Metaphor*. Austin: University of Texas Press, 1982.

———. *Technology as Symptom and Dream*. New York: Routledge, 1989.

Rosen, Stanley. *Plato's Symposium*. New Haven: Yale University Press, 1968.

Sallis, John. *Being and Logos: The Platonic Dialogue*. Pittsburgh: Duquesne University Press, 1975.

Schenk, Ronald. "Bare Bones: The Aesthetics of Arthritis." In *The Body in Analysis*, edited by Nathan Schwartz-Salant and Murray Stein. Wilmette, Illinois: Chiron Publications, 1986.

Stolnitz, Jerome. "Beauty: Some Stages in the History of an Idea." *Journal of the History of Ideas* 22, no. 2 (1961): 185–204.

———. "Beauty." In *The Encyclopedia of Philosophy*, edited by Paul Edwards. New York: Macmillan, 1967.

———. "Of the Origins of 'Aesthetic Disinterestedness'." In *Aesthetics: A Critical Anthology*, edited by George Dickie and R. J. Sclafani. New York: St. Martin's Press, 1977.

Van den Berg, J. H. *The Changing Nature of Man*. New York: W. W. Norton and Co., 1961.

Von Franz, Marie Louise. *A Psychological Interpretation of the Golden Ass of Apuleius*. Irving, Tex.: Spring Publications, 1980.

Weber, Max. *The Protestant Ethic and the Spirit of Capitalism*. Translated by Talcott Parson. New York: Charles Scribners and Sons, 1958.

Wheelwright, Phillip. *Heraclitus*. New York: Atheneum, 1964.

Wilshire, Bruce. *Role Playing and Identity*. Bloomington: Indiana University Press, 1982.

Wind, Edgar. *Pagan Mysteries in the Renaissance*. New York: W. W. Norton and Co., 1968.

Wood, Robert. "Art and the Sacred." In *Listening: Journal of Religion and Culture* 18, no. 1 (Winter 1983).

———. "Immanuel Kant." In *A Path into Metaphysics: Phenomenological, Hermeneutical and Dialogical Studies*. Albany: State University of New York Press, 1990.

———. "Aesthetics in the Kantian Project." Unpublished article.

Zimmerman, Robert L. "Kant: The Aesthetic Judgement." *Journal of Aesthetics and Art Criticism* 21, no. 3 (Spring 1963): 333–44.

# NAME INDEX

Addison, Joseph, 15, 104–5
Alberti, Batista, 95–96
Alexander, Clement of, 75–76
Alhazan, 93
Aphrodite: and appearance, 10, 29, 37–43, 44, 50; Christian degradation of, 74–81; dark, 41–42; as demon, 12–13; as desire, 71; grace, 40–53; as light, 60; as mediator, 51; as soul, 42
Apollo, 120
Arendt, Hanna, 17, 23–24, 64, 72–74, 119, 134–36, 149 n., 150 n.
Aristotle, 149 n., 156 n.
Armstrong, A. Hilary, 10, 46–51
Augustine, Saint, 12, 13, 14, 71–72, 86–89
Auvergne, William of, 92

Bachelard, Gaston, 145
Bacon, Roger, 93
Baumgarten, Alexander, 102
Baxter, Richard, 78
Bernard, Saint, 153 n.
Berry, Patricia, 161 n.
Berry-Hillman, Patricia, 161 n.
Blake, William, 16, 119, 122–23, 132, 142
Boethius, 88
Bonaventure, Saint, 153 n.
Botticelli, Sandro, 38, 40, 82, 91
Brunelleschi, Filippo, 93–95
Burke, Edmund, 15, 105–6

Cassirer, Ernst, 91, 158 n.
Clark, Kenneth, 38–40, 81–82
Constantine, 74
Constantine V, 77
Corbin, Henri, 39, 148
Cornford, F. M., 88
Cusa, Nicholas of, 46, 52–53

Dante, 60, 152 n.

Descartes, Rene, 15, 18, 100, 101, 145
Dionysius the Areopagite, 12, 61–63, 65, 67; and archetype 154 n.
Dionysus, 120
Diotima, 48, 57, 66, 152 n.
Dodds, E. R., 72–74
du Berry, Duc, 153 n.
Duns Scotus, John, 154 n.
Durer, Albrecht 90, 98–99

Eco, Umberto, 153–54 n.
Edgerton, Samuel, 14, 96
Epictetus, 73–74
Eusebios, 74

Ficino, Marsilio, 10, 12, 29; and contemplative life, 135; and light, 62–63; and love, 55–56; and order, 45–46, 51; and spirit, 71; and unity, 66
Freud, Sigmund, 16, 50, 123–25, 152 n.
Friedrich, Paul, 37
Frye, Northrup, 122

Gadamer, Hans-George, 12, 17, 21, 30; and beauty, 26, 56, 60–61, 150 n., the good and the beautiful, 66; and Kant, 108; and knowledge, 147 and language, 137; and *theoria*, 138
Galen, 83, 96, 126
Galileo, 100
Gasché, Rudolph, 101, 115
Goethe, Johann Wolfgang von, 68
Goodheart, William, 139–40
Gregory the Great, 74
Grosseteste, Robert, 92

Heidegger, Martin, 148; and beauty, 122, 152 n., and Being, 66–67; and image, 26; and Kant, 15, 110, 115; and knowledge, 11, 58–60; and language, 137, 152 n.; and subjectivism, 101
Heraclitus, 44, 51, 66, 128, 151 n.

# SUBJECT INDEX